RESEARCH AND PERSPECTIVES IN ENDOCRINE INTERACTIONS

Springer

Berlin
Heidelberg
New York
Barcelona
Hong Kong
London
Milan
Paris
Tokyo

C. Kordon   I. Robinson
J. Hanoune   R. Dantzer   Y. Christen (Eds.)

Brain Somatic Cross-Talk and the Central Control of Metabolism

With 46 Figures and 2 Tables

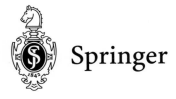 Springer

Kordon, Claude,
Institut Necker
156, rue de Vaugirard
75015 Paris, France
e-mail: kordon@necker.fr

Robinson, Iain
Division of Molecular
Neuroendocrinology
National Institute for Medical Research
The Ridgeway, Mill Hill
London NW7 1AA, U.K.
Tel.: 44 208 913 8575
Fax: 44 208 906 4477

Hanoune, Jacques
Service Endocrinologie
Hôpital Henri Mondor – INSERM U.99
51, Av Mal Lattre de Tassigny
94010 Creteil
Tel.: 01 49 81 35 30, Fax: 01 48 98 09 08
e-mail: hanoune@im3.inserm.fr

Dantzer, Robert
INSERM U.394
Rue Camille Saint Säens
33077 Bordeaux Cedex
Tel.: 05 57 57 37 25, Fax: 05 56 98 90 29
e-mail:
robert.dantzer@bordeaux.inserm.fr

Christen, Yves, Ph. D.
Fondation IPSEN
Pour la Recherche Thérapeutique
24, rue Erlanger
75781 Paris Cedex 16
France
e-mail:
yves.christen@beaufour-ipsen.com

ISBN 3-540-00090-9 Springer-Verlag Berlin Heidelberg New York

Cataloging-in-Publication Data applied for
Bibliographic information published by Die Deutsche Bibliothek
Die Deutsche Bibliothek lists this publication in the Deutsche Nationalbibliografie;
detailed bibliographic data is available in the Internet at <http://dnb.ddb.de>.

Springer-Verlag a member of BertelsmannSpringer
Science + Business Media GmbH

http://www.springer.de

© Springer-Verlag Berlin Heidelberg 2003
Printed in Germany

Production: PRO EDIT GmbH, 69126 Heidelberg, Germany
Cover design: design & production, 69121 Heidelberg, Germany
Typesetting and reproduction of the figures: AM-productions GmbH, 69168 Wiesloch, Germany
Printed on acid-free paper   27/3135Re – 5 4 3 2 1 0

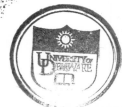

Contents

List of authors

Aubert, Michel L.
Hôpital des Enfants, HUGs, 6, rue Willy-Donzé, 1211 Geneva 14, Switzerland,
Tel. 41 22-382 45 68, Fax 41 22-347 59 79,
e-mail: Michel.Aubert@medecine.unige.ch

Bassant, Marie-Helene
U549 INSERM, 2ter rue d'Alésia, 75014 Paris, France

Betancourt, Lorena
Huffington Center on Aging and Department of Molecular and Cellular Biology,
Baylor College of Medicine, One Baylor Plaza, M320, Houston, TX 77030, USA

Bluet-Pajot, Marie-Therese
U549 INSERM, 2ter rue d'Alésia, 75014 Paris, France

Boutin, Philippe
CNRS-Institute of Biology of Lille, Pasteur Institute of Lille,
1 rue Calmette BP245, 59016 Lille, France, Tel. 33-320 87 79 54,
Fax 33-320 87 72 29

Bowers, Cyril Y.
Department of Medicine, Division of Endocrinology,
Tulane University Medical Center, New Orleans, Louisiana 70112-2699, USA

Caminos, J. E.
Department of Physiology, Endocrine Aera Complejo Hospitalario,
University of Santiago, Santiago de Compostela, 15705, Spain

Casanueva, F.
Department of Physiology, Endocrine Aera Complejo Hospitalario,
University of Santiago, Santiago de Compostela, 15705, Spain

Casteilla, L.
UMR 5018, CNRS-UPS, IFR 31, CHU Rangueil, 1 Avenue Jean Poulhés,
31054 Toulouse Cedex, France

Clifton, Donald K.
Department of Obstetrics and Gynecology, University of Washington
School of Medecine, Seattle, WA 98195-7290, USA

Cousin, B.
UMR 5018, CNRS-UPS, IFR 31, CHU Ranguei, 1 Avenue Jean Poulhés,
31054 Toulouse Cedex, France

Dardennes, Roland
CMME, IFR Broca Ste-Anne, 2ter rue d'Alésia, 75014 Paris, France

Dickson, Suzanne, L.
Department of Physiology, University of Cambridge, Downing Street,
Cambridge CB2 3EG, UK, Tel. 44 1223 333 895, Fax 44 1223 333 840,
e-mail: Sld20@cam.ac.uk

Diéguez, C.
Department of Physiology, Endocrine Aera Complejo Hospitalario,
University of Santiago, Santiago de Compostela, 15705, Spain

Epelbaum, Jacques
Institut National de la Santé et de la Recherche Médicale U549,
IFR Broca-Sainte Anne, 2ter rue d'Alésia, 75014 Paris, France,
Tel. 331-40 78 92 32, Fax 331-45 80 72 93, e-mail: Epelbaum@broca.inserm.fr

Estour, Bruno
Hôpital Bellevue, 14, boulevard Pasteur, St. Etienne, France

Foulon, Christine
CMME, IFR Broca Ste-Anne, 2ter rue d'Alésia, 75014 Paris, France

Froguel, Philippe
CNRS-Institute of Biology of Lille, Pasteur Institute of Lille,
1 rue Calmette BP245, 59016 Lille, France and Barts and The London Genome
Centre, London, UK

García, M. C.
Department of Physiology, Endocrine Aera Complejo Hospitalario,
University of Santiago, Santiago de Compostela, 15705, Spain,
Tel. 0034-981 582658, Fax 0034-981 574145, e-mail: Fscadio@usc.es

Gualillo, O.
Department of Physiology, Endocrine Aera Complejo Hospitalario,
University of Santiago, Santiago de Compostela, 15705, Spain

Hewson, Adrian K.
Department of Physiology, University of Cambridge, Downing Street,
Cambridge CB2 3EG, UK

Jansson, John-Olov
Department of Physiology, University of Cambridge, Downing Street,
Cambridge CB2 3EG, UK

Junien, Claudine
INSERM U383, "Genetique, Chromosome et Cancer", Université Paris V,
Hôpital Necker – Enfants Malades, 149 Rue de Sévres, 75015 Paris, France

Juréus, Anders
Department of Physiology and Biophysics, University of Washington
School of Medecine, Seattle, WA 98195-7290, USA

Kordon, Claude
U549 INSERM, 2ter rue d'Alésia, 75014 Paris, France

Laharrague, P.
UMR 5018, CNRS-UPS, IFR 31, CHU Rangueil, 1 Avenue Jean Poulhés,
31054 Toulouse Cedex, France

Lall, Sabrina
Department of Physiology, University of Cambridge, Downing Street,
Cambridge CB2 3EG, UK

Leloup, C.
UMR 5018, CNRS-UPS, IFR 31, CHU Rangueil, 1 Avenue Jean Poulhés,
31054 Toulouse Cedex, France

Lopez, M.
Department of Physiology, Endocrine Aera Complejo Hospitalario,
University of Santiago, Santiago de Compostela, 15705, Spain

Lorsignol, A.
UMR 5018, CNRS-UPS, IFR 31, CHU Rangueil, 1 Avenue Jean Poulhés,
31054 Toulouse Cedex, France

Nogueiras, R.
Department of Physiology, Endocrine Aera Complejo Hospitalario,
University of Santiago, Santiago de Compostela, 15705, Spain

Pénicaud, L.
UMR 5018, CNRS-UPS, IFR 31, CHU Rangueil, 1 Avenue Jean Poulhés,
31054 Toulouse Cedex, France

Pierroz, Dominique D.
Division of Biology of Growth and Development, Department of Pediatrics,
School of Medicine, 6, rue Willy-Donzé, 1211 Geneva 14, Switzerland

Poindessous-Jazat, Frederique
U549 INSERM, 2ter rue d'Alésia, 75014 Paris, France

Pollmächer, Thomas
Max Planck Institute of Psychiatry, Krapelinstr. 10, 80804 München, Germany

Pralong, François P.
Division of Endocrinology and Metabolism, Department of Medicine,
University School of Medicine, 6, rue Willy-Donzé, 1011 Lausanne, Switzerland

Raposinho, Paula D.
Division of Biology of Growth and Development, Department of Pediatrics,
School of Medicine, 6, rue Willy-Donzé, 1211 Geneva 14, Switzerland

Rio, Marie Christine
IGBMC, CNRS/INSERM U184/ULP, Parc d'Innovation – BP 163,
67404 Illkirch, France

Señaris, R. M.
Department of Physiology, Endocrine Aera Complejo Hospitalario,
University of Santiago, Santiago de Compostela, 15705, Spain

Shimomura, Iichiro
Department of Frontier Bioscience, Graduate School of Frontier Bioscience, and
Department of Medicine and Pathophysiology, Graduate School of Medicine,
Osaka University, 2-2 Yamadaoka, Suita, Osaka 565-0871, Japan,
Tel. 81-6-6879 3270/3272, Fax 81-6-6879 3279, e-mail: Ichi@fbs.osaka-u.ac.jp

Smith, Roy G.
Huffington Center on Aging and Department of Molecular and Cellular Biology,
Baylor College of Medicine, One Baylor Plaza, M320, Houston, TX 77030, USA,
Tel. 713-798 3837, Fax 713-798 1610, e-mail: Rsmith@bcm.tmc.edu

Steiner, Robert A.
Departments of Physiology and Biophysics, Obstetrics and Gynecology,
Room – G-402, University of Washington School of Medicine, Seattle,
WA 98195-7290, USA, Tel. 206 543 87 12, Fax 206 685 06 19,
e-mail: steiner@u.washington.edu

Sudre, Béatrice
Division of Biology of Growth and Development, Department of Pediatrics,
School of Medicine, 6, rue Willy-Donzé, 1211 Geneva 14, Switzerland

Sun, Yuxiang
Huffington Center on Aging and Department of Molecular and Cellular Biology,
Baylor College of Medicine, One Baylor Plaza, M320, Houston, TX 77030, USA

Tannenbaum, Gloria S.
Neuropeptide Physiology Laboratory, McGill University-Montreal Children's
Hospital Research Institute, 2300 Tupper Street, Montreal, Québec H3H 1P3,
Canada, Tel. 514 412-4400, 22753, Fax 514 412 4331,
e-mail: Gloria.tannenbaum@mcgill.ca

Tolle, Virginie
U549 INSERM, 2ter rue d'Alésia, 75014 Paris, France

Tomasetto, Catherine
IGBMC, CNRS/INSERM U184/ULP, Parc d'Innovation – BP 163,
67404 ILLKIRCH, France

Tung, Loraine Y. C.
Department of Physiology, University of Cambridge, Downing Street,
Cambridge CB2 3EG, UK

Vauthay, Delphine
Division of Biology of Growth and Development, Department of Pediatrics,
School of Medicine, 1211 Geneva 14, Switzerland

Zizzari, Philippe
U549 INSERM, 2ter rue d'Alésia, 75014 Paris, France

Introduction

Integrative Control of Feeding, Metabolism, Growth and Reproduction: A Multicentric Dialogue Between Soma and Neuronal Networks

Iain CAF Robinson, Claude Kordon and Yves Christen

This book summarizes presentations made at the Conference on *Brain Somatic Cross Talk and the Central Control of Metabolism,* organised in Paris by the Fondation IPSEN on January 28, 2002. The scope of the Conference, and consequently of the book, was to provide a state-of-the-art outline of the multifaceted neuronal networks, and the multiple neurotransmitters and neuropeptides they produce, which are intimately involved in the regulation of metabolism and energy balance.

Major players controlling hormonal correlates of *growth* and *reproduction* are growth hormone releasing hormone (GHRH), somatostatin and ghrelin for the former, and gonadotropin releasing hormone (GnRH) for the latter. Leptin is involved in both functions. Orexigenic peptides, such as neuropeptide Y (NPY), or anorexigenic ones such as beta-endorphin and corticotropin releasing hormone (CRH), act as common secretion modulators for both growth and reproductive hormones. They also coordinate inhibition of appetite and of gonadotropin secretion through receptors widely distributed throughout the brain.

As they integrate a large number of environmental and somaesthetic signals, the networks serve the highly selective purpose of adapting *energy consumption* to the *availability of food resources.* They tend to limit growth and reproductive activity when sources of energy are scarce, or when stress or emergency situations make it advisable to spare energy. Reproductive functions, which at some periods of times can be considered as *luxury* activities, can be completely turned off by food deprivation or chronic stress, partly by desynchronising GnR and NPY release from median eminence nerve terminals, an effective way to modulate GnRH-gonadotropin amplification levels.

Similarly, growth is impaired in some higher vertebrates by diet restriction, by induction of anorexia, slowed metabolism and by hypothalamic release of somatostatin to block growth hormone secretion. In lower vertebrates (e.g. reptiles) growth can even be totally interrupted for extended periods of time when food is no longer available. Lowered growth hormone and gonadotropin secretion during extensive physical exercise, or induction of temporary amenorrhea in women exposed for a few days to low partial oxygen pressure conditions, such as those prevailing at high altitudes, are other examples of the subordination of adaptive mechanisms to the overall management of energy resources.

The fine setting of major functions by ghrelin and leptin also takes physiological parameters into account. Ghrelin relays gastric information concerning the status of food processing. It increases in anticipation of meals, has a positive effect on fat stores, and affects sleep parameters – which may be another way to structure indirectly, the schedule of food intake. In addition Ghrelin is sensitive to stressful situations, which have been shown to increase its gastric expression. Leptin monitors the status of lipid stores and metabolic parameters, but can also induce partial restoration of responses to insulin in discrete types of insulin resistance, a promising therapeutic complement discussed in this book. In turn, plasma glucose and insulin can increase leptin transport across the blood brain barrier. Leptin can also interact with ghrelin effects, by lowering cellular responses mediated by Ghrelin receptors; it also interacts with CRH, by limiting its sensitivity to adrenal steroid feed back. The latter effect may account for the correlation observed between leptin levels and depression, opening another fascinating physiopathological perspective on brain/somatic cross-talk.

But several other transmitters also act at various levels of the neuronal networks which control the physiology of reproduction and of growth. Their list has been growing at an impressive pace over the past five years, and the conference could not devote an equal emphasis to all of them. As a rule, they are preferentially responsible for the fine tuning of the networks. To quote only some of the most important ones : catecholamines and oxytocin cooperate in controlling both gonadotropins and growth hormone secretion, but can also stimulate feeding. Galanin and proopiomelanocortin (POMC) derivatives relay information from NPY neurons to reproductive and growth responses. The recently discovered galanin-like peptide (GALP) appears to act as an intermediate between leptin and GnRH. Orexins, melanocortin and the Agouti protein are involved in a complex interplay to modulate food intake behaviour. Cocaine-and-amphetamine-regulated transcript (CART), is involved in food intake and neuroendocrine control, besides playing a role in habituation processes and addiction. Insulin-like growth factor-1 (IGF-1), insulin itself, and finally cytokines as IL1 and IL6 can also signal to neuronal networks coordinating management of energy; obesity for instance develops more slowly in transgenic mice bearing a null mutation of the IL6 receptor. This list is by no means exhaustive – new orphan receptors and their cognate peptide ligands are being identified as we write, not to mention a burgeoning field of non-peptide ligands and their receptors in the CNS, which may well also play a part in this integrative behaviour.

An obvious example is in steroid systems. Synaptic release of most of the above neuropeptides is also dependent upon peripheral hormones as estrogens and glucocorticoid, and to a lesser extent progesterone and testosterone. Exposure to steroid hormones in early perinatal life can induce permanent imprinting of neurotransmission characteristics, thus accounting for the gender-dependent pattern of reproductive and growth-related hormonal and behavioural responses. In the adult, they also account for gender adaptation of energy management to physiological conditions, as puberty, pregnancy or stress, which are accompanied by specific hormonal patterns. Gonadal hormones alter the set point of reproductive and growth hormones and account for the marked gender differences in their regulation. Thyroid hormones act rather as coregulators of environmental coping, while adrenal steroids (and CRH) allow the system to adapt to stressful stimuli, thus participating in the hormonal management of emergency situations. Then there is the role of more local growth factors, which can be released from glial cells under defined stress conditions, also participate in the fine tuning of growth hormone and gonadotropin release by relaying glial-neuronal interactions to the pituitary. They can for instance modulate somato-statin release from the median eminence. Central effects of steroid hormones are mediated by neurons of the network expressing their respective nuclear receptors, but also by direct, non genomic effects on neuronal membranes.

Neuropeptides thus act as switches to target adaptive responses to selected organs as a function of internal and environmental challenges. We must clearly move away from considering these peptide signaling systems in isolation. Specific selection of appropriate reponses to pathophysiological situations depends upon particular combinations of neuropeptides released simultaneously within neuronal networks. Sustained upregulation of discrete combinations of genes can stabilise behavioural and hormonal patterns for the entire life of individuals, as those for instance exposed perinatally to specific feeding conditions. Some reports even suggest that such patterns can be transmitted from generation to generation, as illustrated in the last chapter of this book, while other chapters contain many examples of the remarkable mechanisms selected by evolution to optimise the management of energy.

Interactions of Growth Hormone Secretagogues with Leptin-Sensitive Brain Networks

S. L. Dickson[1], L. Y. C Tung[1], S. Lall[1], J.-O. Jansson[1], and A. K. Hewson[1]

Summary

The growth hormone secretagogues (GHS) and ghrelin, an endogenous ligand for the cloned GHS receptor, have recently been shown to induce adiposity in rodents. For some time now, we have been investigating the central site and mechanism of action of GHS, mostly in relation to their growth hormone-releasing action. However, it has become clear that these compounds can activate neuropeptide Y-containing neurones and interact with the hypothalamic circuits controlling body weight and appetite. GHS and ghrelin induce adiposity, although the CNS mechanism underlying this effect may not be fully understood. Hypothalamic circuits regulating body weight can be readily identified as they are responsive to circulating satiety factors such as leptin and insulin. Thus, in electrophysiological studies in vitro we have shown that cells excited by GHS tend to be inhibited by leptin administration. Moreover, GHS-responsive cells appear to be direct targets for leptin, as these responses to GHS and leptin can be observed in a preparation in which synaptic transmission is blocked. Using Fos protein expression to quantify neuronal activation, we have also shown that the hypothalamus is more responsive to GHS/ghrelin in 48-hour fasted rats. This increased responsiveness can be reversed by chronic central infusion of either leptin or insulin. Also refeeding for only two hours at the end of a 48-hour fast reverses the increased responsiveness to GHS, suggesting that central responsiveness to GHS can be regulated acutely, perhaps via some aspect of the feeding process or by absorption of nutrients. We conclude that 1) GHS (and ghrelin) interact with hypothalamic circuits controlling body weight, including leptin- and insulin-sensitive circuits and 2) central responsiveness to GHS is altered by circulating satiety factors and by nutritional state.

Growth hormone secretagogues and ghrelin

The term "growth hormone secretagogue" (GHS) refers to a family of synthetic peptides and non-peptides that stimulate growth hormone (GH) secretion (Bowers et al. 1984) by interacting with the cloned GHS receptor, which is present at

---

[1]Department of Physiology, University of Cambridge, Downing Street, Cambridge CB2 3EG, UK

Kordon et al.
Brain Somatic Cross-Talk and the
Central Control of Metabolism
© Springer-Verlag Berlin Heidelberg 2002

pituitary and hypothalamic sites (Howard et al. 1996). Rather unusually, these synthetic ligands had been available for study long before any natural ligands for the GHS receptor had been identified. In 1999, however, the first endogenous ligand was discovered and named "ghrelin" (Kojima et al. 1999), this was soon followed by the discovery that adenosine is also an endogenous ligand for this receptor (Tullin et al. 2000; Smith et al. 2000). Ghrelin is produced by the oxyntic glands of the stomach and intravenous injection of ghrelin increases acid production and gut motility (Masuda et al. 2000). These physiological actions of ghrelin would be expected of a hormone that is released postprandially and it was therefore surprising to discover that circulating ghrelin levels are actually increased in the fasting state rather than the fed state (Tschöp et al. 2000). However, more recently a marked preprandial rise in plasma ghrelin levels has been reported in humans, suggesting a physiological role in meal initiation (Cummings et al. 2001).

Central actions of growth hormone secretagogues

In 1993, we provided the first direct evidence that GHS are centrally active, as they induced increased electrical activity of a sub-population of hypothalamic arcuate nucleus neurones recorded in vivo and also induced expression of Fos protein in cells in this region (Dickson et al. 1993; 1995). Following these findings, we explored the hypothalamic circuits through which these compounds operate. We showed that the majority of arcuate nucleus cells activated are neuroendocrine cells, both in electrophysiological recordings (Dickson et al. 1995) and from neuroanatomical studies showing that arcuate nucleus cells expressing Fos protein following GHS injection project outside of the blood-brain barrier (by retrograde labelling following systemic retrograde tracer injection; Dickson et al. 1996). As expected from their potent GH-releasing activity, a sub-population of the arcuate nucleus cells that are activated by these compounds include the GH-releasing hormone (GHRH) neurones, as reflected by comparing, on consecutive sections, the overlapping distribution of c-fos and GHRH mRNAs (Dickson and Luckman 1997). However, rather unexpectedly in this study, we discovered that about half of the cells expressing c-fos mRNA also express neuropeptide Y (NPY) mRNA.

Neuropeptide Y, synthesized in the hypothalamic arcuate nucleus and released from terminals in the paraventricular nucleus (PVN), is an important pathway involved in the central regulation of food intake. Indeed, direct injection of NPY into the PVN stimulates feeding in rodents (Stanley and Leibowitz 1985). These NPY neurones also contain another orexigenic peptide, agouti-related protein (AgRP; Hahn et al. 1998), an endogenous melanocortin receptor antagonist. Thus, activation of NPY/AgRP cells by GHS may be responsible for the acute feeding effects observed following injection of GHS (Okada et al. 1996) or ghrelin (Tschöp et al. 2000). Consistent with this finding, selective NPY receptor antagonists or immunoneutralisation of AgRP have been shown to suppress GHS-induced feeding (Nakazato et al. 2001; Shintani et al. 2001). Although ghrelin induces quite marked effects to increase NPY and AgRP gene expression (Kamegai et al. 2001), we have not observed increased NPY gene expression following chronic central infusion of synthetic GHS (Bailey et al. 1999). Whilst the majority of arcuate nucleus cells activated following GHS administration appear to project outside the blood-brain barrier (Dickson et al. 1996), we have shown that GHS activate a small population of arcuate cells that project to the PVN (Honda et al. 1999) that are likely to include NPY neurones.

Whilst systemic administration of exogenous ghrelin has been shown to induce activation of cells in the hypothalamic arcuate nucleus (Hewson and Dickson 2000), it remains to be determined whether the active form of gastric ghrelin is present in the circulation in high enough concentrations to influence hypothalamic function. For activity, the ghrelin molecule has been shown to require an octanoyl side chain on Ser^3 in order to bind and activate the GHS receptor (Bednarek et al. 2000), and the extent to which this side chain is cleaved in the circulation is unknown.

Although the stomach is the main source of circulating ghrelin (Kojima et al. 1999; Dornonville de la Cour 2001), gastrectomy only reduces plasma ghrelin concentrations by 65% (Ariyasu et al. 2001). Ghrelin is also produced in lower quantities by other tissues, e.g., pituitary (Korbonits et al. 2001), kidney (Mori et al. 2000), placenta (Gualillo et al. 2001) and bowel (Ariyasu et al. 2001). Ghrelin mRNA has also been detected in the hypothalamus by PCR. It may be present in very low levels, however, as there have not yet been clear demonstrations of ghrelin mRNA in hypothalamus by in situ hybridization.

Growth hormone secretagogues and ghrelin induce adiposity

In addition to the well-documented effects of GHS and ghrelin on the GH axis (for review see Smith et al. 1997), accumulating data suggest that these compounds may also be involved in the regulation of food intake and body composition. Thus, chronic treatment with both ghrelin and the synthetic GHS induces adiposity in rodents (Lall et al. 2001; Tschöp et al. 2000). Indeed, we observed a marked increase in body fat (measure by Dual X-ray Absorpiometry and fat pad dissection) following as little as two weeks of subcutaneous injections of GHS (Lall et al. 2001). Interestingly we found that twice daily injections were more effective for increasing adiposity than continuous infusions (Fig. 1). These effects of GHS to increase body fat were unexpected, as the elevated GH release achieved by GHS administration would be expected to reduce body fat, as GH is a lipolytic hormone. The mechanism underlying the adiposity may not yet be fully understood. Although both central and peripheral ghrelin injections acutely stimulate food intake (Wren et al. 2000), there does not appear to be any dramatic changes in 24-hour food intake (Fig. 2), suggesting that altered feeding may not be a major contributor to the adiposity. Another possibility is that GHS and ghrelin increase adiposity by increasing circulating glucocorticoids, as these are modestly increased during GHS administration in all species studied (Jacks et al. 1994). However, we showed that the increase in body weight gain seen in intact rats injected twice daily with GHS was also seen in adrenalectomised rats given basal glucocorticoid replacement (Fig. 3). Another possibility is that GHS and ghrelin in-

[A] DEXA: BODY FAT AFTER 2 WEEKS REPEATED INJECTIONS

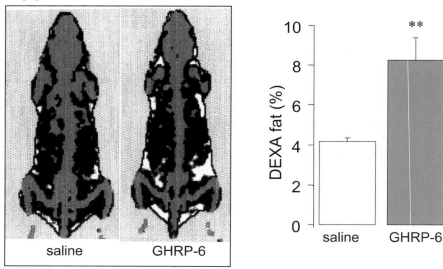

[B] DEXA: BODY FAT AFTER TWO WEEKS INFUSION

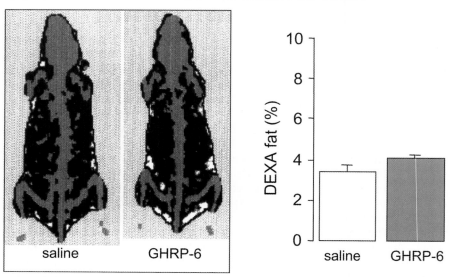

Fig. 1. Changes in body fat visualised by DEXA scans during chronic 15 days of exposure to GHRP-6 or saline vehicle, administered subcutaneously by [A] repeated injections (twice daily) or [B] continuous minipump infusion to mice. Each DEXA image displays a representative normal mouse: white regions of the scans correspond to areas that are >50% fat. The graphs show percentage of DEXA fat measured by DEXA scans after two weeks of GHRP-6 treatment (expressed as the percentage fat-mass relative to the total body area). **p<0.01, compared to saline-treated control mice following a 1-ANOVA with Dunnet's post hoc procedure (n=7-8 for all groups).

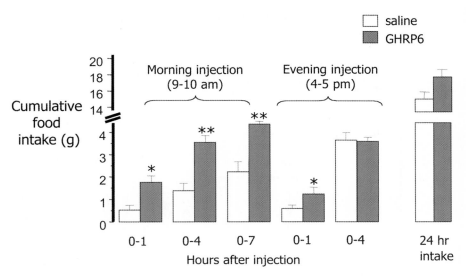

Fig. 2. Cumulative food intake in conscious female rats given a subcutaneous injection of GHRP-6 (250 μg/kg body weight) or saline vehicle, administered in the morning and then again in the afternoon on the same day. Total food intake from time 0 was calculated at 1 hour, 4 and 7 hours (morning only) after each acute injection. Additionally total 24-hour food intake was calculated. N=5–7 per treatment group. *P<0.05, **P<0.01, ANOVA followed by Dunnet's post-hoc test.

crease adiposity by altering nutrient partitioning such that the body spares fat usage, instead using carbohydrates as a preferred energy source (Tschöp et al. 2000).

Ghrelin moonlighting as an anti-leptin signal?

As discussed above, the presence of GHS-R mRNA in over 90% of arcuate nucleus NPY neurones (Willesen et al. 1999), together with the known effects of GHS-R agonists to activate NPY cells and increase NPY gene expression, clearly identify these neurones as a major target for ghrelin/synthetic GHS and may provide a mechanism by which these compounds increase food intake. Arcuate nucleus NPY neurones together with proopiomelanocortin (POMC) cells play a pivotal role in the central regulation of food intake and express receptors for leptin, an adipocyte-derived satiety hormone (for a review see Schwartz et al. 2000). The critical role of leptin in maintaining body weight homeostasis is clearly demonstrated in genetic models of hyperphagia and obesity that result from leptin deficiency (*ob/ob* mice) and leptin resistance (*db/db* mice and *fa/fa* rats). In these models increased expression of arcuate NPY mRNA is observed, which may contribute to the hyperphagia. Replacement of leptin to *ob/ob* mice not only reduces food intake and body weight gain but also suppresses NPY gene expression (Stephens et al. 1995).

Quite clearly ghrelin/GHS and leptin appear to impose opposite effects on arcuate NPY neurones. Interestingly, ghrelin has been proposed to be an anti-leptin signal. Indeed, the ability of leptin to inhibit food intake in rats is abolished when co-administered with ghrelin and, conversely, the stimulatory effect of ghrelin on food intake is reversed by co-administration of leptin (Nakazato et al. 2001; Shintani et al. 2001). Furthermore, the leptin-induced reduction in NPY mRNA ex-

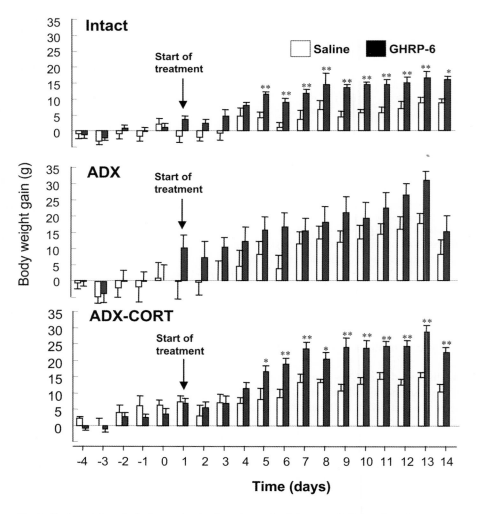

Fig. 3. Body weight gain in intact (top), adrenalectomised (ADX; middle) and corticosterone-replaced adrenalectomised (ADX-CORT) female rats injected twice daily (s.c.) with either saline or GHRP-6 (250 µg/kg body weight). Body weight was measured daily for five days before treatment and then during the 14 days of treatment. Corticosterone was administered orally (25 mg/l in drinking water). N=5-7 per treatment groups. *P<0.05, **P<0.01, ANOVA with Newman-Keuls multiple comparison test.

pression was reversed by co-injection of ghrelin, suggesting a functional antagonism between these two hormones (Shintani et al. 2001). In our own studies we did not see any alteration in the ability of GHS to activate arcuate neurones (i.e., induce Fos protein) in rats infused centrally for seven days with leptin compared to saline-infused controls (Tung et al. 2001). However, using a hypothalamic slice preparation and extracellular electrophysiological recording, we did show that arcuate cells activated by GHS tended to be inhibited by leptin and this inhibition could be observed in preparations in which synaptic transmission was blocked, indicating a direct effect of both compounds on the same cell (Tung et al. 2001). Whilst this extracellular approach does not allow for neurochemical identification of the cell being recorded from, a cell excited by GHS and inhibited by leptin would certainly fit the expected profile of an NPY neurone based on the evidence above. It should be noted, however, that the electrical responses of arcuate nucleus neurones to both GHS and leptin are heterogeneous and that other neuronal populations (e.g., GHRH and POMC) might be expected to respond to both GHS and leptin, albeit with different profiles to NPY neurones.

A picture is emerging of two peripherally produced hormones exerting opposing effects on specific populations of hypothalamic neurones that play a key role in regulating energy intake and energy output. The importance of this interaction as a physiological system involved in either the day-to-day or more long-term control of energy homeostasis remains to be determined.

Increased hypothalamic responsiveness to growth hormone secretagogues and ghrelin in fasting.

Both acute and chronic alterations in energy balance or nutritional status may be relayed to the arcuate nucleus by neuronal pathways or via alterations in the levels of circulating hormones, which may then lead to changes in the activity of NPY and/or POMC neurons. Ghrelin may provide an endocrine link between the stomach and the central circuits involved in the regulation of energy balance, food intake and growth hormone release. There appears to be a fairly major population of cells in the hypothalamic arcuate nucleus that only show increased activity to ghrelin/GHS in rats that have fasted. Thus the number of arcuate nucleus cells detected that express the immediate early genes Fos and Egr-1 in response to GHRP-6/ghrelin injection is about three-fold higher in 48-hour fasted rats than in fed rats (Fig. 4; Luckman et al. 1999; Hewson and Dickson 2000). The most likely explanation is that, in the fed state, hypothalamic responsiveness to GHS/ghrelin is suppressed by circulating levels of absorbed nutrients and/or peripheral satiety signals and that fasting removes this inhibitory influence, allowing more cells to be activated in response to GHS/ghrelin. We have been investigating the possibility that the suppression of circulating leptin and insulin levels brought about by fasting is responsible for the increased hypothalamic responsiveness to ghrelin/GHS (Fig. 5).

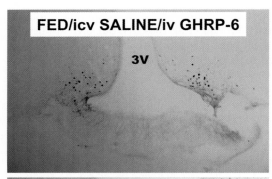

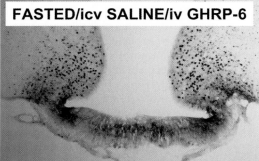

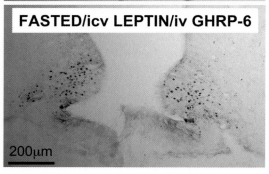

Fig. 4. Fos protein expression in the arcuate nucleus of fed and 48-hour fasted rats given a bolus intravenous injection of 50 μg GHRP-6, a GH secretagogue, at the end of a six-day chronic central infusion (lateral ventricle); 3v, of either saline or leptin (1.2 μg/24 h). The large potentiation of the Fos response observed in fasting was suppressed by central infusion of leptin.

Suppression of feeding and body fat by leptin and insulin

Both leptin and insulin are hypothesized to act as "adiposity signals" to regulate long-term body weight homeostasis via an action on the brain, particularly the arcuate nucleus (Baskin et al. 1999). This model proposes that changes in circulating levels of these hormones in response to alterations in energy homeostasis provide a feedback signal to the hypothalamus to alter food intake and energy utilization accordingly. Receptors for both leptin (Mercer et al. 1996) and insulin (Marks et al. 1990) are expressed in the arcuate nucleus, and central administration of either hormone suppresses food intake and leads to a reduction in body weight. Positive changes in energy balance should lead to increased adiposity and

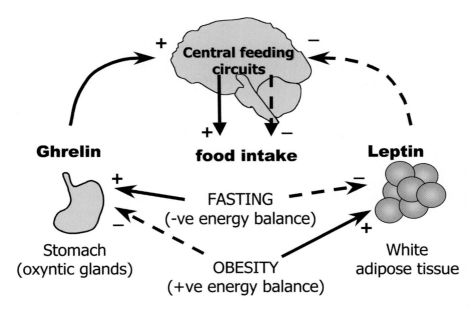

Fig. 5. A hypothetical balancing act between ghrelin, leptin and insulin in the central regulation of food intake and energy homeostasis. As energy stores increase (positive energy balance), circulating levels of leptin and insulin rise and exert a negative feedback signal on hypothalamic feeding circuits while plasma ghrelin levels decrease. In states of negative energy balance, plasma leptin and insulin levels fall, removing the inhibitory effect of these "satiety" hormones on hypothalamic feeding centres. At the same time circulating ghrelin levels are increased and may drive the increased activity of orexigenic pathways (e.g., NPY/AgRP) to stimulate food intake and restore energy homeostasis.

secretion of leptin and insulin, which feed back to the hypothalamus to inhibit food intake and increase energy expenditure. In contrast, a state of negative energy balance such as fasting leads to a marked fall in leptin and insulin levels (Ahima et al. 1996) and to the activation of hypothalamic pathways (e.g., arcuate NPY/AgRP neurones) to increase food intake and restore energy homeostasis (Hahn et al. 1998). Similarly, the absence of these hormones (e.g., *ob/ob* mice, insulin-deficient diabetes melitus, IDDM) or their receptors (e.g., *db/db* mice, neuronal insulin receptor knockouts) results in increased arcuate NPY mRNA expression and hyperphagia (Stephens et al. 1995; Marks et al. 1993; Brüning et al. 2000). Replacement of leptin or insulin to *ob/ob* mice or animals with IDDM respectively, restores NPY mRNA expression to normal and reduces food intake, indicating an inhibitory action of leptin and insulin on arcuate NPY neurones (Stephens et al. 1995; Marks et al. 1993). Moreover, electrophysiological recordings demonstrated a direct inhibitory action of leptin and insulin on a sub-population of arcuate nucleus neurones in lean but not obese (which have primary leptin-resistance and secondary insulin-resistance) Zucker rats (Spanswick et al. 1997 and 2000).

Interactions between ghrelin, leptin and insulin

If the increased hypothalamic responsiveness to GHS in fasted rats is due to the removal of an inhibitory action of leptin and/or insulin, then we should be able to suppress/reverse/prevent the augmented Fos response by replacing leptin or insulin to fasted animals. Initially, however, acute iv or icv bolus administration of leptin to 48-hour fasted rats prior to a bolus iv injection of GHS did not prevent the potentiation of the Fos response (Luckman et al. 1999 and own unpublished observation). This paradigm is complicated somewhat by the fact that leptin administration alone to fasted rats results in the induction of Fos protein in the arcuate nucleus, thus making it impossible to distinguish between cells activated by GHS and those activated by leptin. To circumvent this problem we chose to use a chronic infusion model whereby leptin or insulin was infused directly into the cerebral ventricles for six days and the rats fasted for the last 48-hour of the infusion period. This protocol allowed us to demonstrate that the fasting-induced potentiation of the Fos response to GHS was suppressed in rats receiving central leptin (Fig. 4, Hewson and Dickson 2001) or insulin infusion (not shown) and supports our hypothesis that leptin and insulin exert an inhibitory action on a sub-population of GHS-responsive neurones. We have also found that the Fos response to GHS is significantly greater in obese Zucker rats (which are resistant to the actions of leptin and insulin) compared to their lean, leptin-responsive littermates, which again is in keeping with our hypothesis.

Acute refeeding reverses the increased hypothalamic GHS responsiveness achieved by fasting

While leptin and insulin clearly have an inhibitory action on GHS-responsive cells, other data from our laboratory suggest that the increased hypothalamic responsiveness to GHS in fasting can be prevented by acute re-feeding, apparently independently of circulating leptin and insulin levels. Refeeding for only two hours following a 48-hour fast was associated with suppressed circulating insulin and leptin levels but "normal" glucose levels. Thus, the ability of acute refeeding to prevent the increased neuronal activation induced by GHS in fasted rats may be due to an inhibitory effect of glucose on a sub-population of arcuate neurones. It is also possible that other nutrients may affect hypothalamic neuronal activity independently of insulin or leptin during acute refeeding following a 48-hour fast, and this warrants further investigation. Other possibilities are that stimulation of neural afferents arising in the stomach due to mechanical expansion or release of gut peptides/hormones (e.g., cholecystokinin) achieved during feeding may relay information to the hypothalamus to limit the activation of neurones to exogenously administered GHS.

Summary

A schematic representation of the physiological role of ghrelin is shown in figure 5. While chronic administration of ghrelin/GHS has been shown to induce in rodents adiposity that is in direct contrast to leptin's inhibitory role, current data in humans would suggest ghrelin is unlikely to be a major contributing factor in the pathogenesis of obesity. Plasma levels of ghrelin are significantly lower in obese compared to lean subjects (Tschöp et al. 2001) and were found to decrease in chronically overfed subjects (Ravussin et al. 2001). These data may indicate a compensatory decrease in ghrelin production in response to positive energy balance. In contrast, states such as fasting, exercise-induced negative energy balance and anorexia nervosa are characterized by increased plasma ghrelin levels (Otto et al. 2001; Ravussin et al. 2001). Thus it may be that, in addition to suppression of leptin and insulin levels, conditions of negative energy balance cause an increase in ghrelin secretion to counter further decreases in energy stores and prevent starvation. The findings that the hypothalamic circuits through which GHS (and by extrapolation, ghrelin) act are sensitive to acute perturbations in energy balance (e.g., fasting and refeeding) and subject to inhibitory control by leptin and insulin lend further support to the hypothesis that ghrelin may play a physiological role in the regulation of food intake as well as an adaptive role in the response to negative energy balance.

Acknowledgements

Research supported by the EC Fifth Framework (QLRT-1999-02038). Prof. Claes Olsson and SWEGENE Center for Bio-imaging (CBI) at GothenburgUniversity for excellent help in using DEXA equipment.

References

Ahima RS, Prabakaran D, Mantzoros C, Qu D, Lowell B, Maratos-Flier E, Flier J (1996) Role of leptin in the neuroendocrine response to fasting. Nature 382:250–252

Ariyasu H, Takaya K, Tagami T, Ogawa Y, Hosoda K, Akamizu T, Suda M, Koh T, Natsui K, Toyooka S, Shirakami G, Usui T, Shimatsu A, Doi K, Hosoda H, Kojima M, Kangawa K, Nakao K (2001) Stomach is a major source of circulating ghrelin, and feeding state determines plasma ghrelin-like immunoreactivity levels in humans. J Clin Endocrinol Metab 86:4753–4758

Bailey AR, Giles M, Brown CH, Bull PM, Macdonald LP, Smith LC, Smith RG, Leng G, Dickson SL (1999) Chronic central infusion of growth hormone secretagogues: effects on fos expression and peptide gene expression in the rat arcuate nucleus. Neuroendocrinology 70:83–92

Baskin DG, Figlewicz Lattemann D, Seeley RJ, Woods SC, Porte Jr. D, Schwartz MW (1999) Insulin and leptin: dual adiposity signals to the brain for the regulation of food intake and body weight. Brain Res 848:114–123

Bednarek MA, Feighner SD, Pong SS, McKee KK, Hreniuk DL, Silva MV, Warren VA, Howard AD, Van Der Ploeg LH, Heck JV (2000) Structure-function studies on the new growth hormone-releasing peptide, ghrelin: minimal sequence of ghrelin necessary for activation of growth hormone secretagogue receptor 1a. J Med Chem 43:4370–4376

Bowers CY, Momany FA, Reynolds GA, Hong A (1984) On the in vitro and in vivo activity of a new synthetic hexapeptide that acts on the pituitary to specifically release growth hormone. Endocrinology 114:1537–1545

Brüning JC, Gautam D, Burks DJ, Gillette J, Schubert M, Orban PC, Klein R, Krone W, Müller-Wieland D, Kahn CR (2000) Role of brain insulin receptor in control of body weight and reproduction. Science 289:2122–2125

Cummings DE, Purnell JQ, Frayo RS, Schmidova K, Wisse BE, Weigle DS (2001) A preprandial rise in plasma ghrelin levels suggests a role in meal initiation in humans. Diabetes 50:1–6

Dickson SL, Luckman SM (1997) Induction of *c-fos* mRNA in neuropeptide Y and growth hormone-releasing hormone neurons in the rat arcuate nucleus following systemic injection of the growth hormone secretagogue, GHRP-6. Endocrinology 138:771–777

Dickson SL, Leng G, Robinson ICAF (1993) Systemic administration of growth hormone-releasing peptide activates hypothalamic arcuate neurons. Neuroscience 53:303–306

Dickson SL, Leng G, Dyball REJ, Smith RG (1995) Central actions of peptide and non-peptide growth hormone secretagogues in the rat. Neuroendocrinology 61:36–43

Dickson SL, Doutrelant-Viltart O, Dyball REJ, Leng G (1996) Retrogradely labelled neurosecretory neurones of the rat hypothalamic arcuate nucleus express Fos protein following systemic injection of GH-releasing peptide-6. J Endocrinol 151:323–331

Dornonville de la Cour C, Bjorkqvist M, Sandvik AK, Bakke I, Zhao CM, Chen D, Håkanson R (2001) A-like cells in the rat stomach contain ghrelin and do not operate under gastrin control. Regul Pept 99:141–150

Gualillo O, Caminos JE, Kojima M, Kangawa K, Arvat E, Ghigo E, Casanueva FF, Dieguez C. (2001) Gender and gonadal influences on ghrelin mRNA levels in rat stomach. Eur J Endocrinol 144:687–690

Hahn TM, Breininger JF, Baskin DG, Schwartz MW (1998) Coexpression of Agrp and NPY in fasting-activated hypothalamic neurons. Nature Neurosci 1:271–272

Hewson AK, Dickson SL (2000) Systemic administration of ghrelin induces Fos and Egr-1 proteins in the hypothalamic arcuate nucleus of fasted and fed rats. J Neuroendocrinol. 12:1047–1049

Hewson AK, Dickson SL (2001) Modulation of the arcuate nucleus Fos response to growth hormone-releasing peptide-6 by fasting and leptin (Abstract P3–293). Proceedings of the 83rd Annual Meeting of the Endocrine Society, Denver, CO, p.511

Honda K, Bailey AR, Bull PM, Macdonald LP, Dickson SL, Leng G (1999) An electrophysiological and morphological investigation of the projections of growth hormone-releasing peptide-6-responsive neurons in the rat arcuate nucleus to the median eminence and to the paraventricular nucleus. Neuroscience 90:875–883

Howard AD, Feighner SD, Cully DF, Arena JP, Liberator PA, Rosenblum CI, Hamelin M, Hrenluk DL, Palyha OC, Anderson J, Paress PS, Diaz C, Chou M, Liu KK, McKee KK, Pong S-S, Chaung L-Y, Elbrecht A, Dashkevicz M, Heavens R, Rigby M, Sirinathsinghji DJS, Dean DC, Melillo DG, Patchett AA, Nargund R, Griffin PR, DeMartino JA, Gupta SK, Schaeffer JM, Smith RG, Van der Ploeg LHT (1996) A pituitary gland and hypothalamic receptor that functions in growth hormone release. Science 273: 974–977

Jacks T, Hickey G, Judith F, Taylor J, Chen H, Krupa D, Feeney W, Schoen W, Ok D, Fisher M, et al. (1994) Effects of acute and repeated intravenous administration of L–692,585, a novel non-peptidyl growth hormone secretagogue, on plasma growth hormone, IGF-1, ACTH, cortisol, prolactin, insulin, and thyroxine levels in beagles. J Endocrinol 143:399–406

Kamegai J, Tamura H, Shimizu T, Ishii S, Sugihara H, Wakabayashi I (2001) Chronic central infusion of ghrelin increases hypothalamic neuropeptide Y and Agouti-related protein mRNA levels and body weight in rats. Diabetes 50:2438–43

Kojima M, Kosoda H, Date Y, Nakazato M, Matsuo H, Kangawa K (1999) Ghrelin is a growth-hormone-releasing acylated peptide from stomach. Nature 402:656–660

Korbonits M, Kojima M, Kangawa K, Grossman AB (2001) Presence of ghrelin in normal and adenomatous human pituitary. Endocrine. 14:101–104

Lall S, Tung LYC, Ohlsson C, Jansson J-O, Dickson SL (2001) Growth hormone (GH)-independent stimulation of adiposity by GH secretagogues. Biochem Biophys Res Comm 280:132–138

Luckman SM, Rosenzweig I, Dickson SL (1999) Activation of arcuate nucleus neurones by systemic administration of leptin and growth hormone-releasing peptide-6 in normal and fasted rats. Neuroendocrinology 70: 93–100

Marks JL, Porte Jr. D, Stahl WL, Baskin DG (1990) Localization of insulin receptor mRNA in rat brain by in situ hybridization. Endocrinology 127:3234–3236

Marks JL, Waite K, Li M (1993) Effects of streptozotocin-induced diabetes mellitus and insulin treatment on neuropeptide Y mRNA in the rat hypothalamus. Diabetologia 36:497–502

Masuda Y, Tanaka T, Inomata N, Ohnuma N, Tanaka S, Itoh Z, Hosoda H, Kojima M, Kangawa K (2000) Ghrelin stimulates gastric acid secretion and motility in rats. Biochem Biophys Res Commun. 276:905–908

Mercer JG, Hoggard N, Williams LM, Lawrence CB, Hannah LT, Trayhurn P (1996) Localization of leptin receptor mRNA and the long form splice variant (Ob-Rb) in mouse hypothalamus and adjacent brain regions by in situ hybridization. FEBS Lett. 387:113–116

Mori K, Yoshimoto A, Takaya K, Hosoda K, Ariyasu H, Yahata K, Mukoyama M, Sugawara A, Hosoda H, Kojima M, Kangawa K, Nakao K (2000) Kidney produces a novel acylated peptide, ghrelin. FEBS Lett 486:213–216

Nakazato M, Murakami N, Date Y, Kojima M, Matsuo H, Kangawa K, Matsukura S (2001) A role for ghrelin in the central regulation of feeding. Nature 409:194–198

Okada K, Ishii S, Minami S, Sugihara H, Shibasaki T, Wakabayashi I (1996) Intracerebroventricular administration of the growth hormone-releasing peptide KP-102 increases food intake in free-feeding rats. Endocrinology 137:5155–8

Otto B, Cuntz U, Fruehauf E, Wawarta R, Folwaczny C, Riepl RL, Heiman ML, Lehnert P, Fichter M, Tschop M. (2001) Weight gain decreases elevated plasma ghrelin concentrations of patients with anorexia nervosa. Eur J Endocrinol 145:669–673

Ravussin E, Tschöp M, Morales S, Bouchard C, Heiman ML (2001) Plasma ghrelin concentration and energy balance: overfeeding and negative energy balance studies in twins. J Clin Endocrinol Metab 86:4547–4551

Schwartz MW, Woods SC, Porte D Jr, Seeley RJ, Baskin DG (2000) Central nervous system control of food intake. Nature 404:661–671

Shintani M, Ogawa Y, Ebihara K, Aizawa-Abe M, Miyanaga F, Takaya K, Hayashi T, Inoue G, Hosoda K, Kojima M, Kangawa K, Nakao K (2001) Ghrelin, an endogenous GH secretagogue, is a novel orexigenic peptide that antagonizes leptin action through the activation of hypothalamic neuropeptide Y/Y1 receptor pathway. Diabetes 50:227–232

Smith RG, Van der Ploeg LH, Howard AD, Feighner SD, Cheng K, Hickey GJ, Wyvratt MJ Jr, Fisher MH, Nargund RP, Patchett AA (1997) Peptidomimetic regulation of growth hormone secretion. Endocr Rev 18:621–645

Smith RG, Griffin PR, Xu Y, Smith AG, Liu K, Calacay J, Feighner SD, Pong C, Leong D, Pomes A, Cheng K, Van der Ploeg LH, Howard AD, Schaeffer J, Leonard RJ (2000) Adenosine: a partial agonist of the growth hormone secretagogue receptor. Biochem Biophys Res Commun 276:1306–1313

Spanswick D, Smith MA, Groppi VE, Logan SD, Ashford ML (1997) Leptin inhibits hypothalamic neurons by activation of ATP-sensitive potassium channels. Nature 390:521–525

Spanswick D, Smith MA, Mirshamsi S, Routh VH, Ashford MLJ (2000) Insulin activates ATP-sensitive K+ channels in hypothalamic neurons of lean, but not obese rats. Nature Neurosci 3:757–758

Stanley BG, Leibowitz SF (1985) Neuropeptide Y injected in the paraventricular hypothalamus: a powerful stimulant of feeding behavior. Proc Natl Acad Sci 82:3940–3943

Stephens TW, Basinski M, Bristow PK, Bue-Valleskey JM, Burgett SG, Craft L, Hale J, Hoffmann J, Hsiung HM, Kriauciunas A, MacKellar W, Rosteck Jr PR, Schoner B, Smith D, Tinsley FC, Zhang X-Y, Heiman M (1995) The role of neuropeptide Y in the antiobesity action of the *obese* gene product. Nature 377:530–532

Tschöp M, Smiley DL, Heiman ML (2000) Ghrelin induces adiposity in rodents. Nature 407:908–913

Tullin S, Hansen BS, Ankersen M, Moller J, Von Cappelen KA, Thim L (2000) Adenosine is an agonist of the growth hormone secretagogue receptor. Endocrinology 141:3397–3402

Tung YCL, Hewson AK, Dickson SL (2001) Actions of leptin on growth hormone secretagogue-responsive neurones in the rat hypothalamic arcuate nucleus recorded in vitro. J Neuroendocrinol 13:209–215

Willesen MG, Kristensen P, Rømer J (1999) Co-localization of growth hormone secretagogue receptor and NPY mRNA in the arcuate nucleus of the rat. Neuroendocrinology 70:306–316

Wren AM, Small CJ, Ward HL, Murphy KG, Dakin CL, Taheri S, Kennedy AR, Roberts GH, Morgan DGA, Ghatei MA, Bloom SR (2000) The novel hypothalamic peptide ghrelin stimulates food intake and growth hormone secretion. Endocrinology 141:4325–4328

Leptin and the Neural Circuit Regulating body Weight and Metabolism

M. J. Friedman[1]

Summary

In mammals, a robust physiologic system acts to maintain relative constancy of weight. A key element of this system is leptin. Leptin is an adipocyte hormone that functions as the afferent signal in a negative feedback loop regulating body weight. Leptin also functions as a key link between nutrition and the function of many other physiologic systems. When at their "normal" weight (i.e., normal for that individual), individuals produce a given amount of leptin and in turn maintain a state of energy balance. Weight gain results in an increased plasma leptin level which elicits a biologic response characterized in part by a state of negative energy balance. Weight loss among both lean and obese subjects results in decreased plasma levels of leptin, which leads to a state of positive energy balance and a number of other physiologic responses. Implicit in this construct is that weight is set at different levels among different individuals.

A number of lines of evidence indicate that leptin's principal site of action is in the brain. These data have indicated that leptin acts in part by modulating the activity of efferent signals from the brain that regulate a number of metabolic processes. The nature of this "brain-somatic" cross talk is as yet poorly understood but is likely to have important implications for the pathophysiology and treatment of obesity, diabetes and other metabolic disorders.

Introduction

Substantial advances have been made toward identifying the components of the physiologic system that regulates body weight and the links to nutrition and physiology. Research in this area is at the center of several issues that are of general importance, including 1) obesity, a pressing – some consider the most pressing – health problem in Western and developing countries, 2) the ways in which alterations of nutritional state affect physiology, 3) the role of genes and environment in determining human characteristics, and 4) the molecular basis of behavior

---

[1]Howard Hughes Medical Institute, The Rockefeller University, 1230 York Avenue, Box 305, New York, NY 10021

Kordon et al.
Brain Somatic Cross-Talk and the
Central Control of Metabolism
© Springer-Verlag Berlin Heidelberg 2002

The proposition that obesity is to a large extent the result of biological rather than psychological factors is supported by a plethora of genetic and physiologic data (Kennedy 1953). Twin studies, analyses of familial aggregation and adoption studies all indicate that obesity is the result of major contributions from genetic factors(Calle et al. 1999; Stunkard et al. 1990). Indeed, the hereditability of obesity is roughly equivalent to that of height and exceeds that of many disorders that are generally considered to have a genetic basis. The identity of several of these genes is now known, and in general, they encode the molecular components of the physiological system that regulates body weight and metabolism. Two of the key elements of this system are leptin and its receptor.

Leptin

Leptin is an adipocyte hormone that functions as the afferent signal in a negative feedback loop regulating body weight (Fig. 1). This hormone reports nutritional information (i.e., the size of the organism's energy stores) to the brain and other sites. Leptin circulates as a 16-kilodalton protein in mouse and human plasma but is undetectable in plasma from C57BL/6J *ob/ob* mice (Halaas et al. 1995). *ob/ob*

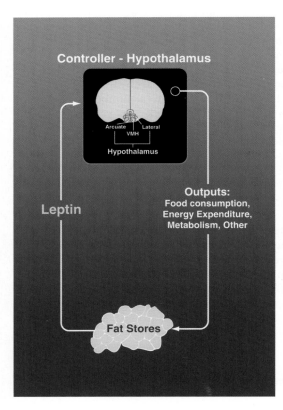

Fig 1. Leptin and the regulation of adipose tissue mass. The cloning of the ob gene and the characterization of leptin have suggested that body fat content is under homeostatic control. The available data suggest that leptin is the afferent signal in a negative feedback loop regulating adipose tissue mass. The level of leptin is positively correlated with differences in body fat. Increasing leptin levels result in negative energy balance (energy expenditure < food intake) whereas decreasing levels lead to positive energy balance (food intake > energy expenditure). These effects maintain constancy of fat cell mass. The available data also suggest that the hypothalamus is an important site of leptin action.

mice are genetically obese as a result of mutations in the leptin gene (Zhang et al. 1994; Coleman 1978). In the absence of leptin, these mutant animals (as well as leptin-deficient humans, see below) never receive the signal that there are adequate fat stores and, in turn, they become hyperphagic and obese.

Leptin is not modified post-translationally because the molecular mass of the native protein is identical to that predicted by the primary sequence (without the signal sequence; Cohen et al. 1996). The plasma level of leptin is highly correlated with adipose tissue mass and falls after weight loss in both humans and mice (Maffei et al. 1995). The levels of protein are increased in several genetic and environmentally induced forms of rodent obesity and in obese humans. Administration of recombinant leptin, either by injection or as a constant subcutaneous infusion to wild type mice, results in a dose-dependent decrease in body weight at incremental increases of plasma leptin levels within the physiologic range (Halaas et al. 1995,1997)

In aggregate, these data establish leptin's role as a hormonal signal in a feedback loop modulating the size of adipose tissue mass and indicate that, to a significant extent, body weight is under endocrine control. However, leptin is not the only afferent signal that regulates food intake and body weight. The systems that control feeding behavior and energy balance appear to be comprised of a short-term and long-term system. The short-term system regulates meal pattern and feeding throughout the day. Previous work has indicated that changes in plasma glucose concentration, body temperature, plasma amino acids, cholecystokinin and other hormones can all modulate meal patterns (Spigelman and Flier 1996). The long-term system balances food intake and energy expenditure and thus plays a dominant role in ultimately regulating the size of the body's energy stores.

Leptin appears to function largely within the longterm system and influences the quantity of food consumed relative to the amount of energy that is expended. Leptin levels do not increase significantly after a meal and it does not, by itself, lead to the termination of a meal (Maffei et al. 1995). These results suggest that leptin is not a classic satiety factor. However, leptin and the other components of the long-term system interact extensively with the components of the short-term system, by modulating the amount of food that is consumed during a meal and/or the likelihood that an organism will miss a meal.

A Broader Role for Leptin

Quantitative changes in plasma leptin concentration elicit a potent biological response. Decreases in plasma leptin levels activate what can be termed a "Response to Starvation," whereas increasing leptin levels illicit a "Response to Obesity" (Fig. 2).The presence of low plasma levels of leptin indicates that there are inadequate amounts of fat (stored energy) and that an adaptive response that would lead to the replenishment of those stores needs to be effected. Several clues concerning the nature of this "Response to Starvation" were provided by detailed analyses of the phenotype of *ob* mice. Leptin- deficient (*ob/ob*) mice manifest myriad endocrine and metabolic abnormalities (Coleman 1978). Many of these derangements, which include decreased body temperature, hyperphagia, de-

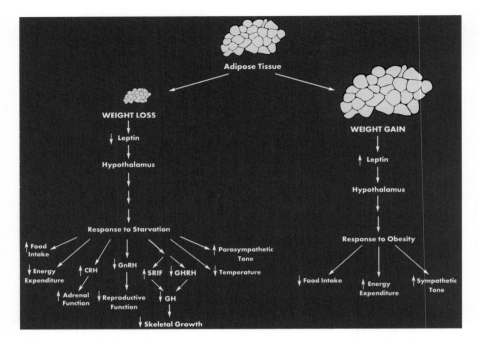

Fig 2. Biologic response to high vs. low leptin levels. Leptin allows the body to maintain constant stores of fat. A loss of body fat (starvation) leads to a decrease in leptin, which in turn leads to a state of positive energy-balance wherein food intake exceeds energy expenditure. This biologic response also includes a pleiotype set of effects on the hypothalamic pituitary axis. Other effects include decreased temperature and an increase of parasympathetic tone. Conversely, an increase in adiposity leads to an increase in the levels of leptin. This response also includes a set of novel effects on fat and glucose metabolism and activation of the sympathetic nervous system.

creased energy expenditure (including activity), immune defects and infertility are also observed in starved animals. This finding has suggested that, in the absence of leptin, *ob/ob* mice exist in a state of perceived starvation and thus exhibit a constellation of signs that are characteristic of the starved state. Indeed, in circumstances where food is readily available, this biological response would be expected to lead to the massive obesity evident in *ob/ob* mice. As predicted, replacement of leptin corrects all of the aforementioned abnormalities of mutant *ob/ob* mice (Halaas et al. 1995).

The possibility that falling plasma leptin levels signal nutrient deprivation is further suggested by the observation that exogenous leptin attenuates the neuroendocrine responses to food restriction (Ahima et al. 1996). Fasted wild-type mice receiving leptin continue to ovulate whereas fasted controls given PBS experience an ovulatory delay of several days. Leptin treatment blunts the changes in circulating thyroid hormone and corticosterone levels that are normally associated with food deprivation (Ahima et al. 1996). Starvation is also associated with decreased immune function, and leptin corrects these abnormalities as well

(Lord 1998). In treated *ob/ob* mice, leptin stimulates proliferation of CD4+ T cells and increases production of cytokines by T-helper-1 cells (Lord 1998). These results indicate that leptin may also be a key link between nutritional state and the immune system.

Leptin is also important in regulating the onset of puberty. Extremely thin women often stop ovulating and abnormally thin adolescent women enter puberty later than their heavier counterparts. These observations have suggested that reproductive potential in women is supposed in the absence of adequate nutritional stores. These findings have further suggested that fat tissue may produce a signal that regulates reproduction (Frisch and McArthur 1974). This factor appears to be leptin. Treatment of mice with leptin accelerates the maturation of the female reproductive tract and leads to an earlier onset of the oestrous cycle and reproductive capacity (Chebab et al. 1997). In humans, a surge in plasma leptin concentration is seen in prepubertal males (Mantzoros et al. 1997). The evidence suggests that sufficient levels of leptin are necessary but not sufficient for the onset of puberty. These studies suggest that leptin modulates reproductive function and provides a direct link between reproduction and the nutritional status of an animal.

These observations led some to speculate that leptin's primary physiological role is to signal nutritional status during periods of food deprivation (Flier and Elmquist 1997). However leptin's physiologic role in preventing weight gain has been confirmed in a number of studies. Lean mice given chronic infusions of leptin lose adipose mass in a dose-dependent fashion at leptin levels within the physiological range (Halaas et al. 1997). These data indicate that increasing leptin levels elicits a "Response to Obesity" and that dynamic changes in plasma leptin concentration act to resist weight change in either direction. The precise nature of this response to obesity is less well understood but is under intense investigation (see below).

The Leptin Receptor and Leptin's Sites of Action

The leptin receptor is a member of the cytokine family of receptors. These receptors have a single transmembrane domain and are generally expressed as monomers or dimers on the cell surface. Ligand binding induces dimerization and/or activation of the receptor and activates signal transduction. Ob-R is predicted to have two separate leptin binding regions and binds leptin with nanomolar affinity (Tartaglia et al. 1995). Five splice forms of the leptin receptor that differ at the carboxy terminus have been identified (Lee et al. 1996). Four of these receptor isoforms are membrane bound whereas Ob-Re encodes a secreted form of the receptor that circulates in plasma (Li et al. 1998).

Mutations that disrupt the leptin receptor have been identified in each of the available strains of diabetic (*db/db*) mice. db/db mice are also genetically obese and manifest a phenotype that is identical to that evident in leptin-deficient *ob/ob* mice. DNA sequence analyses of the available db strains have implicated the Ob-Rb form of the receptor as mediating many, if not all, of leptin's weight-reducing effects. The Ob-Rb form is widely expressed but is enriched in the hypothalamus

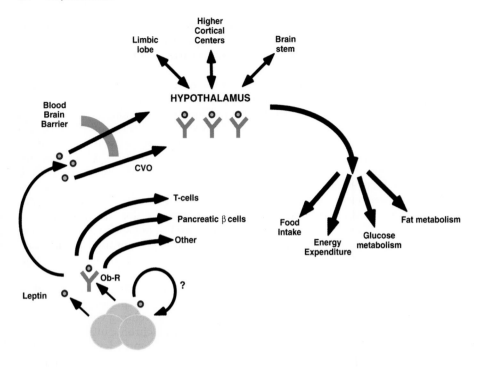

Fig. 3. Adipocyte leptin and the regulation of adipose tissue mass. Leptin is the afferent signal in a negative feedback loop that maintains constancy of adipose tissue mass. Leptin is secreted from adipocytes (bottom left) either as a 16K protein or bound to a soluble form of its receptor (Ob0R). The level of leptin is positively correlated with differences in body fat. Increased leptin results in negative energy balance (energy expenditure > food intake), whereas decreased levels lead to positive energy balance (food intake > energy expenditure). Leptin acts mainly on the hypothalamus (top). Extensive connections exist between the hypothalamus and other brain regions. Leptin acts centrally to decrease food intake and modulate glucose and fat metabolism (right). Peripheral effects on t cells, pancreatic islets and other tissues have also been demonstrated. CVO, circumventricular organ.

(Tartaglia et al. 1995; Lee et al. 1996). These data have suggested that the brain is an important target of leptin action. This possibility is supported by the high potency of leptin when delivered directly into the central nervous system (CNS; Halaas et al. 1997). In addition, leptin modulates the electrical activity of neurons in culture and in slice preparations (Glaum et al. 1996; Cowley et al. 2001).

Leptin also acts on some peripheral cell types and has direct mitogenic effects on CD4+ human T cells (Lord 1998; Fig. 3). It also affects endothelial cells directly and increases angiogenesis, although high doses are required (Sierra-Honegmann et al. 1998). Leptin modulates pancreatic cell function in vivo and also has direct effects on other cell types in vitro, including liver, bone and platelets (Wang et al. 1998). The leptin receptor is widely expressed, though the Ob-Ra (short) form of the receptor predominates in many of these tissues (Lee et al. 1996; Ghilardi et al. 1996; Fei et al. 1997). Although the potency of i.c.v. leptin indicates that direct peripheral effects are not required for weight loss, the full spectrum of leptin's sites of action is not known and could include sites that have not been mentioned.

The function of the short forms of the leptin receptor (Ob-Ra, c, d) is unclear, although it has been suggested that they play a role in mediating the uptake of leptin into the CNS as well as regulating its turnover.

The Neural Circuit Regulating Weight

The available data suggest that the concentration of leptin, glucose and other afferent signals is sensed by groups of neurons in the hypothalamus and other brain regions. During starvation leptin levels fall, thus activating a behavioral, hormonal and metabolic response that is adaptive when energy stores are reduced. Weight gain increases plasma leptin concentration and elicits a different and overlapping response leading to a state of negative energy balance. It is likely that different neurons respond to increasing and/or decreasing leptin levels. In addition, the spectrum of leptin's effects is likely to be complex; as recent studies have indicated, different thresholds exist for several of leptin's effects(Ioffe et al. 1998).

A number of hypothalamic nuclei have been previously implicated in the control of food intake. Thus lesions of the arcuate nucleus, the VMH, DMH and LH perturb body weight and each plays a role in the regulation of food intake or body weight (Choi et al. 1999). Leptin receptors have been localized to each of these hypothalamic nuclei (Fei et al. 1997; Hoggard et al. 1997). The LH and VMH project both within and outside the hypothalamus and modulate activity of the parasympathetic and sympathetic nervous system, respectively (Luiten et al. 1987). The DMH also has inputs to the parasympathetic nervous system and has been implicated in integrating information among the VMH, LH and PVN. The PVN controls secretion of peptides from both the posterior and anterior pituitary and projects to nuclei with sympathetic or parasympathetic afferents (Luiten et al. 1987). The PVN also projects to numerous sites outside of the hypothalamus, including higher centers known to modulate motivational behaviors.

These hypothalamic nuclei express one or more neuropeptides and neurotransmitters that regulate food intake and/or body weight (Spiegelman and Flier 1996). Several lines of evidence have implicated many of these neuropeptides as playing a role in the response to leptin and other nutritional signals. The data are consistent with the possibility that Neuropeptide Y (NPY) and Agouti Related Transcript (ART also known as AGRP) play a role in the response to absent (and possibly low) leptin levels, whereas centrally expressed αMelanocyte Stimulating Hormone (αMSH) and its MC-4 receptor play a role in the response to an increased plasma leptin concentration (Fig. 4; Friedman 1997). Many other neuropeptides, both known and as yet unknown, also play a role in mediating the response to leptin: Melanin concentrating hormone (MCH), a neuropeptide expressed in the lateral hypothalamus, that is increased in *ob/ob* mice and injections of it increase food intake in mice (Qu et al. 1996); CART, a hypothalamic

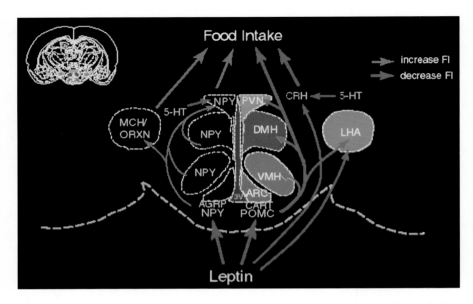

Fig. 4. The neural circuit activated by leptin. In the arcuate nucleus of the hypothalamus the leptin receptor is expressed in at least two different classes of neurons. One class expresses NYP and AGRP, two neuropeptides that increase food intake. Another class expresses POMC, the precursor of αMSH and CART. Both CART and αMSH decrease food intake (FI). The evidence suggests that leptin suppresses the activity of NPY/AGRP neurons and stimulates the activity of POMC/CART neurons. Thus in the absence of leptin the NPY/AGRP neurons are maximally active and food intake is stimulated. In the presence of increased leptin levels the POMC/CART neurons are maximally active and food intake is reduced. When an individual is at his/her stable weight, the activity of these pathways is balanced. The neural mechanisms by which these neurons change food intake are not known. Figure credit: Lex von der Plueg, Merck Pharmaceuticals.

peptide, which is also implicated as playing a role in the response to leptin (Kristensen et al. 1998). CART decreases food intake, CART antibodies increase food intake and its mRNA is increased in *ob/ob* mice; corticotropin-releasing factor (CRF), another factor that is likely to mediate some of leptin's effects, is expressed at high levels in the PVN and in the amygdala, which projects to the LH (Gray et al. 1989; Cummings et al. 1983), and many others. Classical neurotransmitters including serotonin, norepinephrine and dopamine are also known to regulate food intake and all are likely to play a role in the response to leptin.

A fuller understanding of the system that controls weight will also require the identification of the upstream and downstream components of the neural circuit that respond to leptin. Recently a novel system that employs an engineered pseudorabies virus to trace neural circuits has been developed (DeFalco et al. 2001). This vector was successfully used to identify inputs to leptin-responsive neurons in the hypothalamus. The results of studies using this method have shown that a number of brain regions, including pyriform cortex (which processes olfactory information), the amygdala (known to regulate emotional behavior) and cortical regions known to control higher brain functions, can modulate leptin signaling in the hypothalamus (Fig. 5). Studies aimed at understanding the ways in which these multiple relevant inputs are integrated may illuminate the interplay between conscious and unconscious (and other) factors in regulating food intake and body weight. These studies may also have general implications for our understanding of the regulation of a complex behavior.

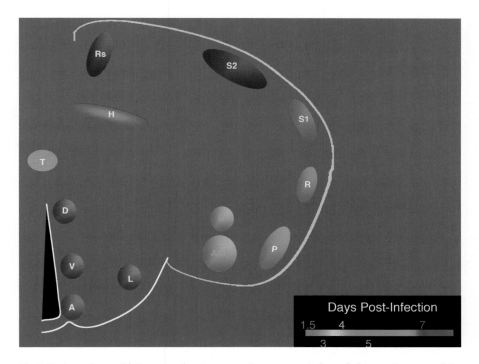

Fig 5. Brain regions with Inputs to leptin-responsive neurons in hypothalamus. A pseusorabies virus that was conditional on cre expression for viral replication and expression of GFP was created. This virus was then injected into the arcuate nucleus of genetically modified mice that express cre in either NPY or leptin receptor-expressing neurons. After infection, the activated virus was propagated retrograde and illuminated neurons that projected, directly or indirectly, to these hypothalamic neurons. Shown are sites where GFP-expressing neurons were observed in forebrain. Time that GFP expression was first noted is indicated by color: red, 1.5 days; orange, 3 days; yellow, 4 days; green, 5 days; blue, 7 days post infection. A, arcuate nucleus; Am, amygdala; B, bed of stria terminalis; D, dorsomedial hypothalamic nucleus; H, hippocampus; L, lateral hypothalamic nucleus; P, pyriform cortex; R, lateral entorhinal and peripheral cortices; Rs, retrosplenial cortices; S1, somatosensory 1 cortex; S2, somatosensory 2 cortex; T, thalamus; V, ventromedial hypothalamic nucleus; (NPY), observed in NPY-Cre mice only; (ObRb), observed in ObRb-IRES-Cre mice only. These results indicate that key hypothalamic neurons integrate leptin's signals and signals from olfactory (pyriform cortex), emotional (amygdala) and higher cortical centers (retrosplenial cortex) and other brain regions.

Efferent Pathways Regulating Metabolism

The evidence indicating that leptin can act centrally to modulate body weight raises the following question: how does the CNS regulate peripheral metabolism in response to differences in leptin and other signals? The effects of leptin on metabolism are distinct from those that are seen after food restriction. While increasing leptin levels lead to fatty acid oxidation and a reduction in adipose tissue mass, leptin deficiency, evident in *ob/ob* mice or mice receiving a leptin anatgonist, is associated with an increase in fat deposition (Coleman 1978; Verploegen et al. 1997). In *ob/ob* mice the rate of lipogenesis is markedly increased, as is the abundance of the RNAs encoding the enzymes that are rate limiting in fatty acid synthesis (Coleman 1978; Loten et al. 1974). It as yet unclear whether the metabolic derangement's of *ob/ob* mice are solely the result of increased food intake or if other factors are also important.

The mechanism by which centrally administered leptin leads to lipolysis and the loss of adipose tissue mass is similarly unclear. It is important to note that increased fatty acid oxidation is not restricted to adipose tissue and that leptin treatment also results in the loss of intracellular lipid in other cell types (Chen et al. 1996). In this and other respects, the available evidence suggests that the metabolic response to leptin is markedly different from the response to reduced food intake. While food restriction (i.e., dieting) leads to the loss of both lean body mass and adipose tissue mass, leptin-induced weight loss is specific for the adipose tissue mass (Halaas et al. 1995, 1997; Levin et al. 1996). Leptin also prevents the reduced energy expenditure normally associated with a decreased food intake (Halaas et al. 1997). Hyperleptinemic animals undergoing a rapid period of weight loss fail to show any rise in serum free fatty acids or ketones (Chen et al. 1996). This finding is in contrast to food-restricted (pair fed) animals, which show a marked rise in serum free fatty acids. Indeed, despite the fact that the respiratory quotient falls after leptin treatment (indicative of fatty acid oxidation), the metabolic fate of stored triglycerides in adipose tissue is unknown (Halaas et al. 1997).

Studies using DNA microarrays have also shown that leptin has a number of novel, indirect (i.e., CNS-mediated) effects on gene expression in adipose tissue (Soukas et al. 2000). Expression monitoring of 6500 genes using oligonucleotide microarrays in wild-type, *ob/ob*, and transgenic mice expressing low levels of leptin revealed that differences in ambient leptin levels have dramatic effects on the phenotype of white adipose tissue. These data identified a large number of genes that are differentially expressed in *ob/ob* mice. To delineate the components of the transcriptional program specifically affected by leptin, the level of the same 6500 genes was monitored in wild type and *ob/ob* mice at various times after leptin treatment or food-restriction. A novel application of k-means clustering identified eight clusters of adipose tissue genes whose expression was different between leptin treatment and food restriction in *ob/ob* mice and 10 such clusters in wild-type experiments. One of the clusters was repressed specifically by leptin in both wild type and *ob/ob* mice and included several genes known to be regulated by SREBP-1/ADD1. It was further shown that leptin decreases the levels of the cleaved, bioactive form of this transcription factor in the cell nucleus (Soukas et al. 2000). These data indicate that leptin's actions on adipose tissue are mediated in part by a decrease in the rate of SREBP cleavage. Since leptin acts on adipose tissue indirectly via its actions on brain, these data suggest that novel neural or metabolic signals are responsible for this cellular response (and others).

Leptin also has novel effects on glucose metabolism. The possibility that leptin modulates glucose metabolism was first suggested in studies of *ob/ob* mice treated with leptin. *ob/ob* mice are diabetic and the severity of the diabetes is dependent on the background strain carrying the mutation (Coleman 1978). In one study, leptin normalized the hyperglycemia and hyperinsulinemia evident in C57BL/6J *ob/ob* mice at doses that did not decrease weight (Pelleymounter et al. 1995). Anti-diabetic effects have also been observed in insulin-deficient rats (Chinookoswong et al. 1999).

Leptin also improves the insulin resistance and hyperglycemia evident in a transgenic mouse line with lipodystrophic (Shimomura et al. 1999). The anti-diabetic effects of leptin in these animals may result from leptin's ability to stimulate lipolysis and fatty acid oxidation in liver, skeletal muscle and other peripheral tissues. Previous studies have indicated that insulin signaling is adversely affected by excess intracellular lipid (McGarry 1992; Randle et al. 1965; Shulman 2000). For example, a selectively increased lipid uptake by liver or muscle leads to decreased insulin action only in that organ (Kim et al. 2001). Thus leptin appears to improve insulin signaling may decreases insulin signaling is not precisely known but may be the result of effects on PKC theta and IRS1 (personal communication) (Shulman 2000). These results could in part explain the frequent association of obesity with insulin resistance, as obesity is associated with increase fat deposition in all cell types, not just adipose tissue.

Recently, Stearoyl CoA Desaturase 1 (SCD-1) has been identified as a key target of the CNS efferent pathways that are activated by leptin (Cohen et al. 2002). SCD-1 introduces a double bond into saturated fatty acids, thus generating monounsaturated fats. Leptin represses this enzyme, and a mutation in the SCD-1 gene, similar to leptin treatment, reduces body weight and increases metabolic rate in both wild type and ob mice. SCD1 deficiency also corrects the fatty liver associated with the ob mutation, further suggesting that drugs that inhibit SCD1 could prove useful in the treatment of obesity and hepatic steatosis. Both of these diseases are of epidemic proportions, and hepatic steatosis is a major cause of end-stage liver disease in the United States and Western Europe. The nature of the CNS efferent signals that regulate SCD-1 gene expression and SREBP cleavage is now under study.

Pathogenesis of Obesity

In principle, alterations in body weight could be the result of abnormalities in the production of leptin, the cells that receive leptin's signal, or the efferent pathways that effect changes in weight. The pathogenesis of obesity can be inferred in a general way by measurement of the plasma leptin levels (Fig. 6). An increase in plasma levels suggests that obesity is the result of leptin resistance. A low or normal plasma concentration of leptin in the context of obesity suggests decreased

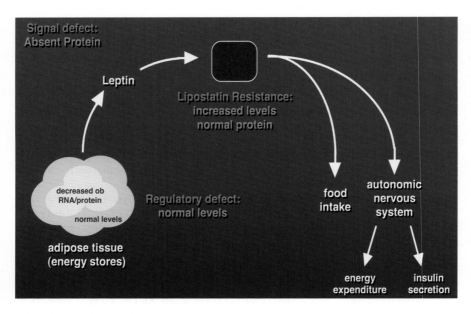

Fig. 6. Pathogenesis of obesity. There are three general ways in which alterations of the leptin regulatory loop could lead to obesity: 1, failure to produce leptin, as occurs in ob/ob mice, would result in obesity, as would 2, inappropriately low leptin secretion for a given fat mass. In the latter case, the fat mass would expand until "normal" leptin levels are reached, resulting in obesity (also see Fig. 5). 3, Finally, obesity could result from relative or obsolete insensitivity to leptin at its site of action. Such resistance would be associated with increased circulating leptin, analogous to the increased insulin levels seen with insulin-resistant diabetes. In general, high plasma leptin levels are evident in obese rodents and humans. In a subset of cases, obesity is associated with normal levels of leptin. Differences in leptin production and leptin sensitivity could be the result of genetic, environmental and psychological factors.

production of leptin. This interpretation is similar to that relating insulin to the pathogenesis of diabetes. However, this designation is quite general, as a great number of hormones as well as genetic, environmental and even psychological factors are likely to influence leptin sensitivity and production.

Plasma leptin levels have been measured in rodents and in humans using both RIA and ELISA (Maffei et al 1995; Considine et al. 1996). In all forms of rodent obesity studied, the obese animals have a higher leptin level than controls (not including *ob/ob* mice; Maffei et al. 1995; Frederich et al. 1995). The data suggest that these forms of animal obesity are the result of leptin resistance. In each of three cases that have been tested, obese animals that are hyperleptinemic are completely or partially resistant to exogenous leptin (Halaas et al. 1997).

DIO (diet-induced obese) mice develop hyperleptinaemia and exhibit a partial response to exogenous leptin. The leptin resistance observed in DIO mice emphasizes the fact that environmental factors can modulate leptin sensitivity. Akr mice (and some other strains) remain lean when fed a standard chow diet but become obese when fed a high fat diet. In contrast, other mouse strains do not become obese when exposed to an identical diet. This finding indicates that the pathogenesis of diet-induced obesity and leptin resistance is the result of an interaction between genetic and environmental factors.

A fuller understanding of the mechanisms by which fat content in the diet modulates weight is likely to be relevant to human obesity. The incidence of obesity increases in many populations in proportion when exposed to a high fat, "Western" diet (Zimmet et al. 1978). How might genes interact with environmental factors to cause obesity? As most people have experienced first hand, exposure to a highly palatable diet often leads to transient weight gain. In most cases, the gained weight is eventually lost. However, it is possible that, in some cases, the induced increase in endogenous leptin level (which accompanies weight gain) leads to a down regulation of the leptin response and a failure to return to the starting weight. If tachyphylaxis to increased leptin is influenced by genetic factors, one might predict that a subset of individuals (and some populations) would be especially susceptible to diet-induced obesity. The observation that animals that express constitutive levels of leptin are insensitive to a high fat diet supports this possibility (unpublished data). However, alternative explanations are possible and additional studies are required. Studies to identify the AKR alleles that predispose to diet-induced obesity may illuminate the underlying mechanism (York et al. 1997; West et al. 1992).

Leptin and Human Obesity

In human subjects, a highly significant correlation between body fat content and plasma leptin concentration has been observed, and obese humans generally have high leptin levels (Maffei et al. 1995; Considine et al. 1996). These data suggest that, in most cases, human obesity is likely to be associated with insensitivity to leptin. However, 5–10 % of obese human subjects have relatively low levels of leptin (Maffei et al. 1995; Considine et al. 1996). Low leptin levels also predispose to weight gain in pre-obese Pima Indians (Ravussin et al. 1997). These data suggest that, in some instances, obesity results from a subnormal secretion rate of leptin from fat.

The basis for leptin resistance in the overwhelming majority of obese, hyperleptinemic human subjects is unknown. Data from studies of animals clearly indicate that this condition is likely to be very heterogeneous and that many factors are likely to influence the activity of the neural circuit that regulates feeding behavior and body weight. It has been suggested that entry of leptin into the CSF may be limiting in some obese subjects, thus leading to leptin resistance (Schwartz et al. 1996;Caro et al. 1996). If true, the development of morbid obesity could result when the plasma leptin levels exceed the capacity of the transport system. Treatment of humans with recombinant leptin has been shown to result in an increase in CSF leptin concentrations (Fujioka et al. 1999). Leptin uptake has been demonstrated in the capillary endothelium of mouse and human brain and is decreased in pre-obese animals (Golden et al. 1997; Banks et al. 1996, 1999). It is not yet known whether this increase in CSF levels after treatment with recombinant leptin is variable among different individuals. It has thus been proposed that transport across the brain capillary endothelium is required for leptin to find its way to its site of action in the brain interstitial space and that Ob-Ra and/or other proteins mediate leptin transport (Golden et al. 1997). Moreover, defects anywhere in this transport pathway could lead to the development of obesity.

Defects in leptin signal transduction could also be important in the development of leptin resistance. Studies of the function of the leptin receptor in vitro have confirmed that Ob-Rb is capable of activating signal transduction (Ghilardi et al. 1996; Tartaglia 1997; White et al. 1997; Bjorbaek et al. 1997). Leptin activates the STAT transcription factor in hypothalamus within 15 minutes of a single intraperitional injection (Vaisse et al. 1996). In vitro studies have indicated that activation of the leptin receptor is dependent on phosphorylation of the JAK2 kinase after ligand binding to an Ob-Rb homodimer. Leptin also leads to the tyrosine phosphorylation of the SHP-2, a phosphotyrosine phosphatase, which in turn decreases both the state of JAK-2 phosphorylation and transcription of a leptin-inducible reporter gene (Carpenter et al. 1998; Li and Friedman 1999). Thus SHP-2 may play a role in shutting off the leptin signal transduction pathway. SOCS-3, a suppressor of JAK signaling, has also been implicated in leptin signal transduction and may also play a role in down regulating the response to leptin (Bjorbaek et al. 1998). Other components of the leptin signal transduction pathway have not yet been identified.

Leptin resistance in humans is likely to be the result of a complex interplay of many factors. In principle, leptin resistance could result from altered activity of any of the aforementioned components of the leptin signal transduction pathway in the cells that respond directly on any cells downstream in this neural circuit. Indeed, leptin's actions are likely to be influenced by psychological factors via connections between the higher cortical centers that modulate an animal's motivational state and neural circuits within the hypothalamus (DeFalco et al. 2001). The neuroanatomic and functional relationships between these brain regions are only now being elucidated.

Mutations Associated With Human Obesity

In almost all cases, obese subjects express at least some leptin. Recently, two cousins born from an extended family have been found to be homozygous for a frame shift mutation in the leptin gene. These individuals do not have any circulating leptin (Montague et al. 1997a). In these two subjects, the mutation is associated with profound obesity, confirming that leptin is of critical importance for the control of body weight in humans. Affected members of a Turkish kindred with a missense mutation in the leptin gene have reduced leptin levels and also manifest extreme obesity and amennorhea, which further suggests that leptin also plays a role in modulating reproductive function (Strobel et al. 1998). Similar conclusions were reached in studies of three massively obese members of a French family carrying mutations in the leptin receptor (Clement et al. 1998). These three studies also indicate that, apart from severe obesity and abnormalities of reproductive function, the other abnormalities identifiable in *ob/ob and db/db* mice, such as hypertcortisolemia, cold intolerance and severe diabetes, are not necessarily apparent.

Mutations in other genes are also associated with human obesity. Available evidence suggests that as many as 1–2 % of morbidly obese humans have mutations in the human MC-4 Receptor (Yeo et al. 1998). In these cases, the obesity is inherited in a dominant mutation, indicating that a 50 % decrease in αMSH signaling can have important effects on body weight. A recent report showed linkage of POMC and other loci on human chromosome 2 to leptin levels and, to a lesser extent, BMI in a population of Mexican Americans (Comuzzie et al. 1997). Proopio melano cortin (POMC) is the precursor of αMSH. Variation at this locus may contribute to leptin resistance. The importance of MSH signaling is also illustrated by the development of obesity in two individuals with mutations in the POMC gene (Krude et al. 1998). Obesity has also been observed in a woman with a mutation in the PC-1 gene (Jackson et al. 1997). PC-1 is a protease that is known to cleave neuropeptide precursors and thus serves a similar function to CPE, the gene that is mutant in *fat/fat* mice (Naggert et al. 1995).

The association of massive obesity with mutations in leptin and its receptor in humans, while rare, confirms their importance in regulating body weight. This assertion is supported by data from early clinical trials with leptin in humans (see below). However, mutations in these genes, and POMC, PC-1 and the MC4 Receptor are relatively rare. Thus the pathogenesis of most human obesity is unknown. It is likely that some of the genes responsible for human obesity in the general population will at some level modulate either leptin secretion or leptin sensitivity. Both genetic and physiological studies will be required to confirm this prediction.

Leptin and the Treatment of Human Obesity and Diabetes

A recent prospective epidemiologic study of more than one million individuals has confirmed that obesity is an independent risk factor for increased mortality (Calle et al. 1999). This finding amplifies the need for efficacious and safe means for treating this disorder. The health risk of obesity is greatly diminished when even modest amounts of weight (i.e., 5 % of total weight) are lost (Blackburn 1995; Sjostrom et al. 1997). This decreased risk is the result of a marked improvement in the diabetic, hypertensive, and cardiovascular status of obese subjects affected by these conditions (Blackburn 1995). Dieting, by itself, is only rarely effective for the long-term maintenance of weight loss, emphasizing the need for additional therapies (Wadden 1993). Clearly an important indication for leptin treatment would be the management of the co-morbidities associated with obesity, such as diabetes (see below).

Early studies of leptin treatment in the general population have demonstrated that four weeks of leptin injections are safe and cause small but significant weight loss in lean and obese subjects compared to placebo ($p < 0.02$; unpublished observation). Treatment of eight obese subjects for a total of six months resulted in an average weight loss of 7.1 kg in a group receiving 0.3 mg/kg leptin vs. 1.7 kg in a group receiving placebo. Some of the subjects in this latter group lost substantial amounts of weight while others did not. This limited study suggests that leptin could ultimately emerge as an effective therapy for at least some obese subjects, although studies of more patients are clearly required (Heymsfield et al. 1999).

Leptin treatment has proven to be more effective in treating patients with either complete or partial leptin deficiency. Leptin treatment is clearly effective for treating obese patients with mutations in the leptin gene (Farooqi et al. 1999; Montague et al. 1997b). In addition to reducing food intake and weight and body fat content, the hormone stimulated cycling of gonadotrophins in one of the pre-pubescent children and also corrected his immune defects. The efficacy of treatment with exogenous leptin in these subjects confirms that leptin plays a physiological role in regulating weight in humans and also establishes a link between leptin signaling and reproductive capacity (Farooqi et al. 1999).

In addition to congenital leptin deficiency, other previously unappreciated clinical syndromes resulting from leptin deficiency have recently been identified. Human lipodystrophy, the congenital or acquired loss of adipose tissue, is associated with leptin deficiency and is characterized by a grossly enlarged fatty liver and a severe insulin-resistant form of diabetes. Leptin treatment has also been shown to correct the diabetes, insulin resistance and fatty liver associated with this condition in humans (Oral et al. 2002). These findings further emphasize the need to elucidate the CNS signaling pathways that regulate insulin sensitivity. The data also suggest that leptin could prove useful in other settings of insulin resistance, provided that the treated individual is leptin-sensitive (i.e., has a low endogenous leptin level).

Conclusion

Studies of the physiological system that regulates weight have identified several molecules that have potential as therapeutic targets. Leptin or leptin agonists may be of use for the treatment of obesity and other disorders such as lipodystrophy. αMSH agonists and NPY antagonists are also in development. The fact that patients with MC4R mutations exhibit an obese phenotype makes αMSH agonists particularly attractive as a potential therapy antagonists would also be of potential benefit in light of the lean phenotype of MCH knockout mice. It is highly likely that, as additional components of the system that regulates weight are identified, new therapeutic modalities will be developed. An important area in this regard is the identification of the efferent CNS signals that are modulated by leptin and in turn regulate metabolism. Whether or not new therapies emerge, the identification of leptin and its receptors has provided an intellectual framework in which to consider the regulation of food intake and body weight, the pathogenesis of obesity and other nutritional disorders and the links between nutrition and physiology.

Acknowledgments

The author would like to thank Susan Korres for expert assistance in preparing this manuscript and Alex Soukas for helpful comments. This work was supported by a grant from NIH/NIDDK (J.M.F.) and in part by a NIH MSTP grant GM07739 (J.L.H.).

References

Ahima RS, Prabakaran D, Mantzoros C, Qu D, Lowell B, Maratos-Flier E, Flier JS (1996) Role of leptin in the neuroendocrine response to fasting. Nature 382: 250–252.

Banks W, DiPalma C, Farrell C (1999) Impaired transport of leptin across the blood-brain barrier in obesity. Peptides, 20 : 1341–1345

Banks WA, Kastin AJ, Huang W, Jaspan JB, Maness LM (1996) Leptin enters the brain by a saturable system independent of insulin. Peptides 17:305–311.

Bjorbaek C, Elmquist JK, Frantz JD, Shoelson SE, Flier JS (1998) Identification of SOC-3 as a potential mediator of central leptin resistance. Mol Cell 1: 619–625.

Bjorbaek C, Uotani S, da Silva B, Flier JS (1997) Divergent signaling capacities of the long and short isoforms of the leptin receptor. J Biol Chem 272: 32686–32695.

Blackburn G (1995) Effect of degree of weight loss on health benefits. Obesity Res 3 (Suppl. 2): 211s–216s.

Calle E, Thun MJ, Petrelli JM, Rodriguez C, Heath CW Jr (1999) Body-mass index and mortality in a prospective cohort of U.S. adults. N Engl J Med 341:1097–1105.

Caro J, Kolaczynski JW, Nyce MR, Ohannesian JP, Opentanova I, Goldman WH, Lynn RB, Zhang PL, Sinha MK, Considine RV (1996) Decreased cerebrospinal-fluid/serum leptin ratio in obesity: a possible mechanism for leptin resistance. Lancet 348:159–161.

Carpenter LR, Farruggella TJ, Symes A, Karow ML, Yancopoulos GD, Stahl N (1998) Enhancing leptin response by preventing SH2-containing phosphatase 2 interaction with ob receptor. Proc Natl Acad Sci USA 95:6061–6066.

Chehab FF, Chehab FF, Mounzih K, Lu R, Lim ME (1997) Early onset of reproductive function in normal female mice treated with leptin. Science 275:88–90.

Chen G, Koyama K, Yuan X, Lee Y, Zhou YT, O'Doherty R, Newgard CB, Unger RH (1996) Disappearance of body fat in normal rats induced by adenovirus-mediated leptin gene therapy. Proc Natl Acad Sci USA 93:14795–14799.

Chinookoswong N, Wang J, Shi Z (1999) Leptin restores euglycemia and normalizes glucose turnover in insulin-deficient diabetes in the rat. Diabetes 48:1487–1492.

Choi SJ, Sparks R, Clay M, Dallman MF (1999) Rats with hyporthalamic obesity are insensitive to central leptin injections. Endocrinology 140:4426–4433.

Clement K, Vaisse C, Lahlou N, Cabrol S, Pelloux V, Cassuto D, Gourmelen M, Dina C, Chambaz J, Lacorte JM, Basdevant A, Bougneres P, Lebouc Y, Froguel P, Guy-Grand B (1998) A mutation in the human leptin receptor gene causes obesity and pituitary dysfunction. Nature 392:398–401.

Cohen L, Halaas JL, Friedman JM, Chait BT, Bennett L, Chang D, Hecht R, Collins F (1996) Characterization of endogenous human leptin. Nature 382:589.

Cohen P, Miyazaki M, Socci ND, Hagge-Greenberg A, Liedtke W, Soukas AA, Sharma R, Hudgins LC, Ntambi JM, Friedman JM (2002) Role for stearoyl-CoA desaturase-1 in leptin mediated weight loss. Science 297:240–243.

Coleman DL (1978) Obese and diabetes: two mutant genes causing diabetes-obesity syndromes in mice. Diabetologia 14:141–148.

Comuzzie AG, Hixson JE, Almasy L, Mitchell BD, Mahaney MC, Dyer TD, Stern MP, MacCluer JW, Blangero J (1997) A major quantitative trait locus determining serum leptin levels and fat mass is located on human chromosome 2. Nature Genet 15:273–276.

Considine RV, Considine EL, Williams CJ, Hyde TM, Caro JF (1996) The hypothalamic leptin receptor in humans: identification of incidental sequence polymorphisms and absence of the db/db mouse and fa/fa rat mutations. Diabetes 45: 992–994.

Cowley M, Smart JL, Rubinstein M, Cerdan MG, Diano S, Horvath TL, Cone RD, Low MJ (2001) Leptin increases the activity of arcuate POMC neurons by two mechanism. Science, in press

Cummings S, Elde R, Ells J, Lindall A (1983) Corticotropin-releasing factor immunoreactivity is widely distributed within the central nervous system of the rat: an immunohistochemical study. J Neurosci 3:1355–1368.

DeFalco J, Tomishima M, Liu H, Zhao C, Cai X, Marth JD, Enquist L, Friedman JM (2001) Virus-assisted mapping of neural inputs to a feeding center in the hypothalamus. Science 291:2608–2613.

Farooqi I, Jebb SA, Langmack G, Lawrence E, Cheetham CH, Prentice AM, Hughes IA, McCamish MA, O'Rahilly S (1999) Effects of recombinant leptin theraphy in a child with congenital leptin deficiency. N Engl J Med 341: 879–884.

Fei H, Okano HJ, Li C, Lee GH, Zhao C, Darnell R, Friedman JM (1997) Anatomic localization of alternatively spliced leptin receptors (Ob-R) in mouse brain and other tissues. Prod. Natl. Acad. Sci USA 94:7001–7005.

Flier JS, Elmquist JK (1997) Energetic pursuit of leptin function. Nature Biol 15:20–21.

Frederich RC, Hamann A, Anderson S, Lollmann B, Lowell BB, Flier JS (1995) Leptin levels reflect body lipid content in mice: evidence for diet-induced resistance to leptin action. Nature Med 1:1311–1314.

Friedman JM (1997), The alphabet of weight control. Nature385: 119–120.

Frisch RE, McArthur JW(1974) Menstrual cycles: fatness as a determinant of minimum weight for height necessary for their maintenance or onset. Science 185:949–951.

Fujioka K, Patane J, Lubina J, Lau D (1999) CSF leptin levels after exogenous administration of recombinant methionyl human leptin. JAMA 282:1517–1518.

Ghilardi N, Ziegler S, Wiestner A, Stoffel R, Heim MH, Skoda RC (1996), Defective STAT signaling by the leptin receptor in diabetic mice. Proc Natl Acad Sci USA 93: 6231–6235.

Glaum SR, Hara M, Bindokas VP, Lee CC, Polonsky KS, Bell GI, Miller RJ (1996) Leptin, the obese gene product, rapidly modulates synaptic transmission in the hypothalamus. Mol Pharmacol 50 :230–235.

Golden PL, Maccagnan TJ, Pardridge WM (1997) Human blood-brain barrier leptin receptor. Binding and endocytosis in isolated human brain microvessels. J Clin Invest 99:1418.

Gray TS, Carney ME, Magnuson DJ (1989) Direct projects from the central amygdaloid nucleus to the hypothalamic paraventricular nucleus: Possible role in stress-induced adrenocorticotropin release. Neuroendocrinology 50:433–446.

Halaa JL, Gajiwala KS, Maffei M, Cohen SL, Chait BT, Rabinowitz D, Lallone RL, Burley SK, Friedman JM (1995) Weight-reducing effects of the plasma protein encoded by the obese gene. Science 269:543–546.

Halaas JL, Boozer C, Blair-West J, Fidahusein N, Denton DA, Friedman JM (1997) Physiological response to long-term peripheral and central leptin infusion in lean and obese mice. Proc Natl Acad Sci USA 94:8878–8883.

Heymsfiel S, Greenberg AS, Fujioka K, Dixon RM, Kushner R, Hunt T, Lubina JA, Patane J, Self B, Hunt P, McCamish M (1999) Recombinant leptin for weight loss in obese and lean adults. JAMA 282:1568–1575.

Hoggard N, Mercer JG, Rayner DV, Moar K, Trayhurn P, Williams LM (1997) Localization of leptin receptor mRNA splice variants in murine peripheral tissues by RT-PCR and in situ hybridization. Biochem Biophys Res Commun. 232:383–387.

Ioffe E, Moon B, Connolly E, Friedman JM (1998) Abnormal regulation of the leptin gene in the pathogenesis of obesity. Proc Natl Acad Sci USA 95:11852–11857.

Jackso RS, Creemers JW, Ohagi S, Raffin-Sanson ML, Sanders L, Montague CT, Hutton JC, O'Rahilly S (1997)Obesity and impaired prophormone processing associated with mutations in the human prohormone convertase 1 gene. Nature Genet 16:303–306.

Kennedy GC (1953) The role of depot fat in the hypothalamic control of food intake in the rat. Proc Roy Soc (London) (B) 140: 578–592.

Kim JK, Fillmore JJ, Chen Y, Yu C, Moore IK, Pypaert M, Lutz EP, Kako Y, Velez-Carrasco W, Goldberg IJ, Breslow JL, Shulman GI (2001) Tissue specific overexpression of lipoprotein lipase causes tissue specific insulin resistance. Proc Natl Acad Sci USA 98: 7522–7527.

Kristensen P, Judge ME, Thim L, Ribel U, Christjansen KN, Wulff BS, Clausen JT, Jensen PB, Madsen OD, Vrang N, Larsen PJ, Hastrup S (1998) Hypothalamic CART is a new anorectic peptide regulated by leptin. Nature 393:72–76.

Krude H, Biebermann H, Luck W, Horn R, Brabant G, Gruters A (1998), Severe early-onset obesity, adrenal insufficiency and red hair pigmentation caused by POMC mutations in humans. Nature Genet. 19:155.

Lee GH, Proenca R, Montez JM, Carroll KM, Darvishzadeh JG, Lee JI, Friedman JM (1996) Abnormal splicing of the leptin receptor in diabetic mice. Nature 379:632–635.

Levin N, Nelson C, Gurney A, Vandlen R, de Sauvage F (1996) Decreased food intake does not completely account for adiposity reduction after ob protein infusion. Proc Natl Acad Sci USA 93:1726–1730.

Li C, Friedman J (1999) Leptin receptor activation of SH2 domain protein tyrosone phosphatase 2 modulates ob receptor signal transduction. Proc Natl. Acad Sci USA 96:9677–9682.

Li C, Ioffe E, Fidahusein N, Connolly E, Friedman JM (1998) Absence of soluable leptin receptor in plasma from dbPas/dbPas and other db/db mice. J Biol Chem 273:10078–10082.

Lord G (1998) Leptin modulates the T-cell immune response and reverses starvation induced immunosuppression. Nature 394:897–891.

Loten EG, Rabinovitch A, Jeanrenaud B (1974) In vivo studies in obese hyperglycaemic (ob/ob) mice: possible role of hyperinsulinaemia. Diabetologia10:45–52.

Luiten PGM, Horst GJ, Steffens AB (1987) The hyothalamus, intrinsic connections and outflow pathways to the endocrine system in relation to the control of feeding and metabolism. Progress Neurobiol 28:1–54.

Maffei M, Halaas J, Ravussin E, Pratley RE, Lee GH, Zhang Y, Fei H, Kim S, Lallone R, Ranganathan S, Kern PA, Friedman JM (1995) Leptin levels in human and rodent: Measurement of plasma leptin and ob RNA in obese and weight-reduced subjects. Nature Med 1:1155–1161.

Mantzoros CS, Flier JS, Rogol AD (1997) A longitudinal assessment of hormonal and physical alterations during normal puberty in boys. Rising leptin levels may signal the onset of puberty. J Clin Endocrinol Metab 82:1066–1070.

McGarry JD (1992) What if Minkowski had been ageusic? An alternative angle on diabetes. Science 258:766–770.

Montague CT, Farooqi IS, Whitehead JP, Soos MA, Rau H, Wareham NJ, Sewter CP, Digby JE, Mohammed SN, Hurst JA, Cheetham CH, Earley AR, Barnett AH, Prins JB, O'Rahilly S (1997a) Congenital leptin deficiency is associated with severe early-onset obesity in humans. Nature 387: 903–908.

Montague CT, Prins JB, Sanders L, Digby JE, O'Rahilly S (1997b) Depot- and sex-specific differences in human leptin mRNA expression: implications for the control of regional fat distribution. Diabetes, 46:342–347.

Naggert JK, Fricker LD, Varlamov O, Nishina PM, Rouille Y, Steiner DF, Carroll RJ, Paigen BJ, Leiter EH (1995) Hyperproinsulinaemia in obese fat/fat mice associated with a carboxypeptidase E mutation which reduces enzyme activity. Nature Genet10:135–142.

Oral EA, Simha V, Ruiz E, Andewelt A, Premkumar A, Snell P, Wagner AJ, DePaoli AM, Reitman ML, Taylor SI, Gorden P, Garg A (2002) Leptin-replacement therapy for lipodystrophy. N Engl J Med 346:570–578.

Pelleymounter MA, Cullen MJ, Baker MB, Hecht R, Winters D, Boone T, Collins F (1995) Effects of the obese gene product on body weight regulation in ob/ob mice. Science 269:540–543.

Qu D, Ludwig DS, Gammeltoft S, Piper M, Pelleymounter MA, Cullen MJ, Mathes WF, Przypek R, Kanarek R, Maratos-Flier E (1996) A role for melanin-concentrating hormone in the central regulation of feeding behavior. Nature 380:243–247.

Randle PJ, Garland PB, Newsholme EA, Hales CN (1965) The glucose fatty-acid cycle in obesity and maturity onset diabetes mellitus. Ann NY Acad Sci 131:324–333.

Ravussi E, Pratley RE, Maffei M, Wang H, Friedman JM, Bennett PH, Bogardus C (1997) Relatively low plasma leptin concentrations precede weight gain in Pima Indians. Nature Med 3:238–240.

Schwartz MW, Peskind E, Raskind M, Boyko EJ, Porte D Jr (1996) Cerebrospinal fluid leptin levels: relationship to plasma levels and to adiposity in humans. Nature Med 2:589–593.

Shimomura I, Hammer RE, Ikemoto S, Brown MS, Goldstein JL (1999) Leptin reverses insulin resistance and diabetes mellitus in mice with congenital lipodystrophy. Nature 401:73–76.

Shulman GI (2000) Cellular mechanisms of insulin resistance. J Clin Invest 106:171–176.

Sierra-Honigmann M, Nath AK, Murakami C, Garcia-Cardena G, Papapetropoulos A, Sessa WC, Madge LA, Schechner JS, Schwabb MB, Polverini PJ, Flores-Riveros JR (1998) Biologic action of leptin as an angiogenic factor. Science 281:1683–1686.

Sjostrom CD, Lissne L, Sjostrom L (1997) Relationships between changes in body compostition and changes in cardiovascular risk factors: The SOS Intervention Study. Obesity Res 5: 519–530.

Soukas A, Cohen P, Socci ND, Friedman JM (2000) Leptin-specific patterns of gene expression in white adipose tissue. Genes Dev 14: 963–980.

Spiegelman BM, Flier JS (1996) Adipogenesis and obesity: rounding out the big picture. Cell 87: 377–389.

Strobel A, Issad T, Camoin L, Ozata M, Strosberg AD (1998) A leptin missense mutation associated with hypogonadism and morbid obesity. Nature Genet 18:213–215.

Stunkard AJ, Stunkard AJ, Harris JR, Pedersen NL, McClearn GE (1990) The body-mass index of twins who have been reared apart. N Engl J Med, 322:1483–1487.

Tartaglia LA (1997) The leptin receptor. J BiolChem 272: 6093–6096.

Tartaglia LA, Dembski M, Weng X, Deng N, Culpepper J, Devos R, Richards GJ, Campfield LA, Clark FT, Deeds J, Muir C, Sanker S, Moriarty A, Moore KJ, Smutko JS, Mays GG, Woolf EA, Monroe CA, Tepper RI (1995) Identification and expression cloning of a leptin receptor, OB-R. Cell 83:1263–1271.

Vaisse C, Halaas JL, Horvath CM, Darnell JE Jr, Stoffel M, Friedman JM (1996) Leptin activation of Stat3 in the hypothalamus of wild-type and ob/ob mice but not db/db mice. Nature Genet 14: 95–97.

Verploegen S, Plaetinck G, Devos R, Van der Heyden J, Guisez Y (1997) A human leptin mutant induces weight gain in normal mice. FEBS Lett 405:237–240.

Wadden TA (1993) Treatment of obesity by moderate and severe caloric restriction. Results of clinical research trials. Ann Intern Med 119: 688–693.

Wang MY, Koyama K, Shimabukuro M, Mangelsdorf D, Newgard CB, Unger RH (1998) OB-Rb gene transfer to leptin-resistant islets reverses diabetogenic phenotype. Proc Natl Acad Sci USA 95:714–718.

West DB, Boozer CN, Moody DL, Atkinson RL (1992) Obesity induced by a high fat diet in nine strains of inbred mice. Am J Physiol 262:R1025–R1032.

White DW, Kuropatwinski KK, Devos R, Baumann H, Tartaglia LA (1997) Leptin receptor (OB-R) signaling. Cytoplasmic domain mutational analysis and evidence for receptor homo-oligomerization. J Biol Chem 272:4065–4071.

Yeo G, Farooqi IS, Aminian S, Halsall DJ, Stanhope RG, O'Rahilly S (1998) A frameshift mutation in MC4R associated with dominatly inherited human obesity. Nature Genet 20:111–112.

York B, Lei K,West DB (1997) Inherited non-autosomal effects on body fat in F2 mice derived from an AKR/J x SWR/J cross. Mann Genome 8:726–730.

Zhang Y, Proenca R, Maffei M, Barone M, Leopold L, Friedman JM (1994) Positional cloning of the mouse obese gene and its human homologue. Nature 372:425–432.

Zimmet P, Arblaster M, Thoma K (1978) The effect of westernization on native populations. Studies on a Micronesian community with a high diabetes prevalence. Australian N Z J Med 8:141–146.

Role of the Growth Hormone Secretagogue Receptor in the Central Nervous System

R. G. Smith[1], L. Betancourt[1], and Y. Sun[1]

Summary

Aging is accompanied by a decline in the amplitude of the release of hormones, neurotransmitters and neuropeptides. These changes are associated with alterations in metabolism resulting in increases in deposition of visceral fat at the expense of muscle. My laboratory is investigating the underlying mechanism of this declining activity of the central nervous system (CNS) and related metabolic alterations. Our objective is to reverse, delay or prevent these changes. We focused on the age-dependent attenuation of pulsatile growth hormone release as a paradigm because of the known anabolic effects of GH. Accordingly, we characterized and expression cloned a new orphan G-protein coupled receptor, the growth hormone secretagogue receptor (GHS-R), which regulates the amplitude of GH pulsatility. In situ hybridization showed that the GHS-R was expressed in CNS regions controlling hormone release from the pituitary gland and in regions enriched in dopaminergic and serotonergic neurons, all of which are known to be involved in metabolism as well as in control of appetite. The physiological relevance of the GHS-R has been confirmed by identification of two natural ligands, ghrelin and adenosine. Interestingly, these endogenous ligands are reported to increase appetite. Besides rejuvenating the GH axis, the GHS-R ligands activate a subset of NPY neurons, and it has been speculated that this property explains the stimulation of feeding behavior. To determine how closely ghrelin mimics the properties of MK-0677, the synthetic ligand for GHS-R, we constructed site-directed mutants of the GHS-R and compared their activity when treated with the two ligands. The results showed that ghrelin occupies a different activation pocket than that occupied by MK-0677. Although administration of ghrelin mimics many of the in vivo effects of MK-0677, ghrelin appears to be less GHS-R selective, suggesting that ghrelin may act through a GHS-R subtype. Studies with GHS-R -/- and ghrelin -/- mice will establish whether ghrelin and MK-0677 act on different GHS-R subtypes and whether the metabolic and orexigenic effects are mediated through different signaling pathways.

[1]Huffington Center on Aging and Department of Molecular and Cellular Biology, Baylor College of Medicine, One Baylor Plaza, M320, Houston, Texas 77030, USA

Kordon et al.
Brain Somatic Cross-Talk and the
Central Control of Metabolism
© Springer-Verlag Berlin Heidelberg 2002

Introduction

Our focus is to define the physiological role of the growth hormone secretagogue receptor (GHS-R) in the central nervous system (CNS). Here, we have selected aspects of GHS-R biology that relate to changes in metabolism that occur during aging. Indeed, the earliest signs of aging are increased fat deposition and reduced muscle mass. Such metabolic-based changes are a health concern because of increased risk of developing "Syndrome X" (type II diabetes, hyperlipidemia, atherosclerosis and hypertension). Metabolism is governed by interactions between the endocrine and nervous systems and this interdependence makes it difficult to make a clear distinction between neuronal and hormonal regulation.

Biological Rhythms and Metabolism

Aging of the neuroendocrine system is manifested by reduced pulse amplitude and increased irregularity in the periodicity of hormone, neuropeptide, and neurotransmitter release. For example, erratic firing of reduced amplitude has been described in neurons of the suprachiasmatic nucleus (SCN) during aging in rats (Satinoff et al. 1993). Age-related changes in circadian rhythms have been linked to the development of obesity and insulin resistance. In old rats, with age-associated increases in insulin resistance and body fat, modification of their daily rhythms of endogenous corticosterone and prolactin restores the young metabolic phenotype (Cincotta et al. 1993). This was accomplished by administering the hormones at times of the day to mimic the profile observed in young rats. Thus, changes in circadian endocrine rhythms are associated with age-related modifications in carbohydrate and lipid metabolism. Re-establishing the rhythms by appropriately timed hormone replacement restores the young phenotype, emphasizing the physiological importance of circadian rhythmicity.

Alterations in hypothalamic function cause endocrine changes that result in altered metabolism. To identify the hypothalamic areas involved, Bernardis et al. lesioned the dorsal medial nucleus (DMN) and ventromedial nucleus (VMN; Bernardis and Davis 1996). Ablation of the DMN impaired growth and reduced body fat. Glucose and lipid metabolism remained normal. In contrast, ablation of the VMN increased body fat, glucose intolerance and hyperlipidemia. The VMN is a target for leptin, and leptin resistance accompanies aging (Wang et al. 2001). Adiposity and serum leptin levels increase with age in male Brown Norway rats. When serum leptin levels are modified through fasting, hypothalamic neuropeptide Y (NPY) mRNA changes reciprocally in young rats, but not in older rats, which is consistent with impairment of leptin regulation of NPY. When leptin was infused into ad libitum fed young and old rats for seven days, food consumption decreased by 50 % in young rats and 20 % in aged rats (Scarpace et al. 2000). Control rats were then pair-fed the food consumed by leptin-treated rats and oxygen consumption was compared. There was a 24 % increase in oxygen consumption in the young leptin-treated rats. By contrast, no changes in oxygen consumption were measurable in the aged rats. Leptin treatment of young rats produced an almost 50 % decrease in hypothalamic NPY mRNA levels, whereas no reduction was observed in old rats. These studies support the speculation that aged rats are less responsive to leptin as a consequence of impaired suppression of hypothalamic NPY synthesis.

A specific increase in visceral fat (VF) is believed to be an important contributing factor for age-associated insulin resistance and the subsequent development of Syndrome X. Caloric restriction (CR) of rats during aging reduces accumulation of VF and prevents insulin resistance. VF also provides a source of the counter-regulatory hormone for glucose homeostasis, corticosterone in rodents and cortisol in humans. This is partly because VF contains high levels of 11β-hydroxysteroid dehydrogenase type 1 (HSD1), the enzyme that converts 11-keto steroids to active glucocorticoids. Surgical removal of VF in rats improves hepatic insulin action and decreases leptin and TNF-alpha gene expression in subcutaneous adipose tissue (Barzilai and Gupta 1999). Administration of leptin selectively decreases VF by about 60 % and inhibits hepatic glucose production by approximately 80 %. Hence, the relationship between an age-related increase in VF and increased insulin resistance might involve the failure of leptin to regulate fat distribution.

The Brown Norway (BN) rat provides a good model for investigating the neuroendocrine basis of metabolic changes (Matsumoto et al. 2000). During aging, primary and secondary testicular failure is associated with blunted circadian rhythms in LH and testosterone, reductions in the hypothalamic levels of GnRH, and increases in insulin and leptin. However, expression of NPY in the arcuate nucleus decreases. Surprisingly, these endocrine changes are accompanied by reduced food intake. However, body weight increases, accompanied by increased peripheral and visceral adiposity with a decrease in lean body mass. If insulin sensitivity is increased, by treating the aged rats with troglitazone, insulin and leptin levels decline. This decline is accompanied by reduction in body fat, increased food intake, and a loss of body weight during fasting. Interestingly, restoring the young metabolic phenotype does not alter NPY gene expression in the arcuate nucleus (Matsumoto et al. 2000). The results of these experiments are consistent with an age-dependent development of insulin and leptin resistance that contributes to deficits in energy and weight regulation.

Adenovirus-mediated leptin gene transfer has been used to study age-related alterations in the metabolic response to leptin in hyperleptinemic 2-month-old and 18-month-old lean wild type Zucker diabetic fatty rats (Wang et al. 2001). Markedly different responses were observed in old versus young rats that were exposed to the elevated levels of leptin produced by the adenovirus. The effects on reducing food intake, body weight and fat were markedly attenuated in 18-month-old compared to 2-month-old rats. Also, the precipitous drop in free fatty acids and triacylglycerol levels observed in the young rats did not occur in the old rats. Metabolic markers, such as acyl CoA oxidase, carnitine palmitoyl transferase 1 and peroxisome-proliferator-receptor-γ, show marked increases in response to leptin in 2-month-old rats, but the magnitude is attenuated in the 18-month-old rats. These results suggest that the observed age-related alterations in leptin sensitivity involve attenuation of the leptin signal transduction pathway. Suppressor of cytokine signaling-3 (SOCS-3) is a component of this pathway, and its expression in the hypothalamus and white fat increases during aging. Therefore, it is tempting to speculate that increased expression of SOCS-3 explains, at least partially, leptin resistance and abnormalities in lipid metabolism in the elderly.

Growth Hormone (GH)

The blood levels of GH decline as we age. Rudman's group administered GH as a bolus injection to elderly men for six months and was the first to report the potential of GH replacement for reversing the metabolic effects observed during aging (Rudman et al. 1990). However, adverse side effects, such as carpal tunnel syndrome and gynecomastia, were evident in about 50 % of the treated subjects (Rudman et al. 1990). It should be noted that this approach to replacing GH by daily injections is pharmacologic and does not mimic physiology, because in all species studied to date GH is episodically released (Jansson et al. 1985; Miller et al. 1982; Steiner et al. 1978).

The importance of the pulsatile profile is illustrated by a comparison of activation of signal transduction pathways and gene expression in the liver following pulsatile versus sustained administration of GH (Ram et al. 1996; ,Davey et al. 1999). In humans, aging produces reduced GH pulse amplitude and a fall in plasma IGF-1 levels (Ho et al. 1987). Based on the known metabolic properties of GH and IGF-1, this probably explains age-associated alterations in metabolism leading to increased fat/lean ratio, decreased muscle strength, reduced exercise tolerance and increased bone loss. Therefore, we hypothesized that GH replacement would prove beneficial. To test this speculation we sought a method that would allow us to restore a youthful pulsatile GH profile in the elderly.

GH Secretagogue Receptor (GHS-R)

We considered the underlying cause of the reduced amplitude of GH pulsatility and sought to correct this deficiency. Only by restoring the GH pulsatility to mimic normal physiology could we accurately evaluate whether rejuvenating the GH axis was beneficial (Smith et al. 1997). We hypothesized that altered pulsatility was caused by a pivotal change(s) in CNS physiology. GH secretion was once thought to be regulated primarily by two hypothalamic hormones, growth hormone releasing hormone (GHRH) and somatostatin (sst). However, synthetic GH-releasing peptides (GHRPs), described by Momany and Bowers, were also shown to stimulate GH release (Bowers 1996; Bowers et al. 1984, 1990; Momany et al. 1981). Subsequently, small molecule mimetics of the GHRPs, such as L-692,429 and MK-0677, were developed that led to the identification of a new receptor and characterization of a signal transduction pathway distinct from that of GHRH (Cheng et al. 1989, 1991; Patchett et al. 1995; Smith et al. 1993). Attempts to characterize the receptor involved were frustrated by the very low abundance of ligand binding sites in the pituitary gland. Following identification of the potent selective ligand MK-0677, high specific activity ^{35}S-MK-0677 (1200 Ci/mmole) was prepared and shown to bind with high affinity (Kd = 200 pM) and limited capacity to membranes isolated from pituitary and hypothalamic tissues (Dean et al.

1996,; Pong et al. 1996). Remarkably, the concentration of binding sites was exceedingly low in both rat pituitary (Bmax = 2 fmol/mg protein) and hypothalamic membranes (Bmax = 6 fmol/mg protein; Smith et al. 1996b). The ligand binding specificity was consistent with the discovery of a new receptor involved in the control of GH release. For example, L-692,429, MK-0677; Fig. 1) and GHRPs, but not GHRH or sst, competitively inhibited ^{35}S-MK-0677 binding (Pong et al. 1996; Smith et al. 1996b). High affinity binding was inhibited non-competitively by GTP-γ-S, suggesting that the receptor was G-protein coupled (Pong et al. 1996). In 1995 we cloned this receptor and showed it was a new, orphan G-protein coupled receptor (GPCR; Howard et al. 1996; Smith et al. 1997). We named it the GH-secretagogue receptor (GHS-R). The GHS-R has been highly conserved across species throughout evolution and is a member of the Class 1 GPCRs but does not belong to any of the known subfamilies of G-protein coupled receptors (Palyha et al. 2000; Smith et al. 1997, 1999).

In situ hybridization studies using selective, non-overlapping radiolabeled oligonucleotides, showed that expression of *GHS-R* is confined to the pituitary gland and brain (Guan et al. 1997). RNase protection assays confirmed the presence of *GHS-R* transcripts in pituitary, hypothalamus and hippocampus. In the rat pituitary gland, in situ hybridization showed that expression of *GHS-R* was confined to the anterior lobe. This finding is consistent with the observation that a fluorescently tagged biotinylated analog of MK-0677 localized selectively to GH-containing cells, and with functional studies showing that GHRP-6 and MK-0677 selectively act on somatotrophs and somatomammotrophs (Smith et al. 1996a, 1997). In the brain, the *GHS-R* is widely expressed (Guan et al. 1997). Intriguingly, in addition to neurons that play a role in the control of GH release, the receptor is expressed in areas that affect circadian rhythms, mood, cognition, memory and learning.

The GHS-R was shown to regulate the release and amplitude of GH pulsatility (Smith et al. 1997). GHS-R agonists reverse the age-related attenuation of GH pulsatility in elderly subjects (>70 years old) to mimic the amplitude of pulsatility of young adults (20-28 years old; Chapman et al. 1996a). To determine whether the age-related decline in GH pulsatility might be causally related to metabolic

Fig. 1. Orally active GHS-R used in clinical trials.

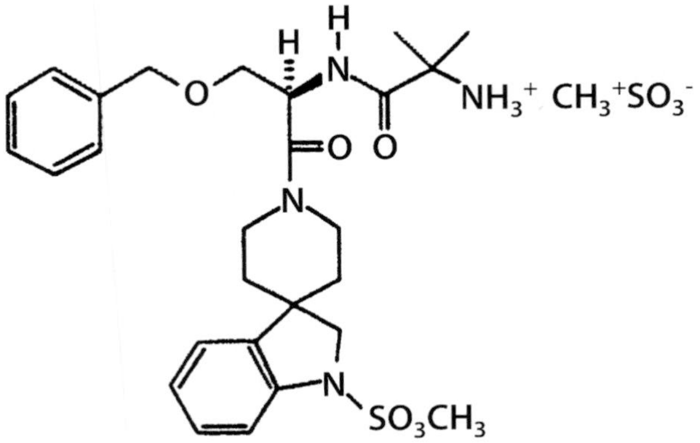

changes, we evaluated whether chronic treatment with the GHS-R ligand MK-0677 would have beneficial effects on body composition, strength and bone turnover. In addition to GH, IGF-1 levels in the elderly were restored to levels typical of young adults; bone turnover and bone mineral density increased, diet-induced catabolism was reversed, body composition improved, and in the frail elderly modest improvements in strength at the shoulder and knee were measured (Chapman et al. 1996a; Murphy et al. 1998, 1999; Svensson et al. 1998; Bach, M. Growth Hormone Society 1996, 1998).

In humans, the long-acting GHS-R ligand, MK-0677, rejuvenates the GH/IGF-1 axis of 70- to 90-year-old subjects to produce GH and IGF-1 levels typical of those of subjects in their late twenties (Chapman et al. 1996b, 1997). Therefore, in the clinic, activators of the GHS-R present a number of potential therapeutic opportunities. Moreover, in contrast to treatment with GH and GHRH, activation of the GHS-R pathway is subject to physiological feedback pathways preventing hyperstimulation of the axis (Smith et al. 1997); hence, in the elderly, the maximum GH and IGF-1 levels attainable are within the normal range of young adults. Most importantly, the well-described effects of the GHRPs and ghrelin on stimulating the release of cortisol and prolactin are not evident during chronic treatment with the longer acting compounds such as MK-0677 (Smith et al. 1997; Chapman et al. 1997). These effects of GHRPs and ghrelin on the cortisol axis probably preclude their use clinically and may explain their associated properties of stimulating appetite and increasing fat deposition (Lawrence et al. 2002; Tschop et al. 2000).

Ghrelin and Adenosine are Endogenous Ligands of the GHS-R

Following cloning of the GHS-R, cell lines that stably expressed the receptor were established and exploited to screen fractions from tissue extracts for an endogenous ligand. The first one disclosed was ghrelin, which is an acylated 28-amino acid peptide that was isolated from the stomach (Kojima et al. 1999). The remarkable feature of this peptide ligand is that octanoylation of a specific serine residue is essential for biological activity. Ghrelin mimics the well-characterized GHS-R synthetic ligands by inducing GH release from pituitary cells in vitro, by stimulating GH release in vivo, and by activating c-fos expression in hypothalamic neurons (Kojima et al. 1999; Hewson and Dickson 2000). It is unclear whether reduced production of ghrelin explains the decline in GH pulse amplitude during aging.

Two other groups identified adenosine in hypothalamic extracts as an endogenous ligand for the GHS-R (Smith et al. 2000; Tullin, et al. 2000). Using HEK293aeq17 cells expressing the GHS-R as an assay for agonist activity, adenosine behaves as a partial agonist (Smith et al. 2000). However, adenosine was also claimed to be a full agonist (Tullin et al. 2000). Adenosine fails to induce secretion of GH from cultured pituitary cells, but in common with ghrelin, adenosine increases food intake (Tullin et al. 2000). Adenosine concentrations in the brain are sufficient to activate the GHS-R ($EC_{50,}$ 2 µM) (Ferre et al. 1997; Premont et al. 1977). In contrast, according to the results of in vitro studies with the cloned GHS-R, it is unclear whether the concentration of free ghrelin in the blood

Ghrelin

Adenosine

OC(CH₂)₆CH₃

GSSFLSPEHQKAQQRKESKKPPAKLQPR

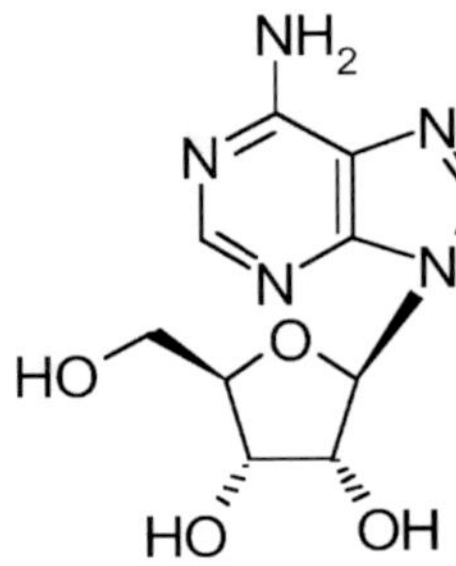

Fig. 2. Endogenous ligands of the GHS-R.

reaches sufficiently high levels to activate the GHS-R in vivo. Perhaps the physiological target for ghrelin is a GHS-R subtype rather than the GHS-R cloned by the Merck group (Howard et al. 1996). Therefore, in spite of the fact that adenosine does not stimulate GH release from isolated pituitary cells, more experiments are needed before ruling out a physiologically important role for adenosine on GHS-R expressed in the brain (Smith et al. 2000).

The potential importance of adenosine as a ligand for the GHS-R in the brain is consistent with the integrative effect of adenosine on dopamine and GABA regulated pathways (Ferre et al. 1997; Ongini and Fredholm 1996; Premont et al. 1977). Adenosine, produced in the pituitary gland, increases tyrosine hydroxylase in hypothalamic cells and stimulates secretion of catecholamines by dopaminergic neurons (Porter et al. 1990, 1991, 1995). During aging there is a decline in the capacity of neurons to secrete dopamine (Hoffman and Sladek 1980; Kish et al. 1992; ThyagaRajan et al. 1995; Yamagami et al. 1992; Yurek et al. 1998); therefore, age-related reductions in dopamine secretion may be a consequence of reduced levels of adenosine (Colao et al. 1999). In old rats, L-dopa administration restores the amplitude of GH release to that of young rats (Sonntag et al. 1982), similar to what is observed with the GHS-R ligand MK-0677 in elderly human subjects (Chapman et al. 1996a). Moreover, both L-dopa and GHS-R ligands increase GHRH levels (Chihara et al. 1986; Fletcher et al. 1996; Guillaume et al. 1994). While MK-0677 does not bind to dopamine receptors, the GHS-R is expressed on dopaminergic neurons (Guan et al. 1997; Smith et al. 1999). Therefore one could speculate that activation of the GHS-R, either by endogenous adenosine or MK-0677, induces dopamine release from hypothalamic neurons. The dopamine then stimulates GHRH release, resulting in increased GH pulse amplitude. Thus, it would be predicted that age-related declines in dopamine and adenosine resulting in attenuation of pulsatile GH release could be rescued by treatment with MK-0677.

Indirect Evidence for GHS-R Subtypes

A series of reports shows that administration of the GHS-R peptide agonist hexarelin is cardioprotective (De Gennaro Colonna et al. 1997a, b; Rossoni et al. 1999; Tivesten et al. 2000). Recently, chronic administration of ghrelin was shown to improve left ventricular dysfunction and attenuate development of cardiac cachexia in rats with heart failure (Nagaya et al. 2001b). In support of a direct role on cardiovascular function, ^{125}I-ghrelin was found to bind with high affinity (Kd = 0.43 nM) to human and rat heart and vasculature (Katugampola et al. 2001). However, interpretation of these data is complicated because the expression of GHS-R in the heart could only be detected using RT-PCR and the levels are extraordinarily low (Hewson and Dickson 2000). It is unlikely that the high affinity binding of ^{125}I-ghrelin involves the GHS-R. In rat pituitary gland the concentration of the GHS-R is 2 fmole/mg membrane protein, and based on a comparison of the intensity of RT-PCR signals from mRNA from pituitary gland and heart, the concentration in the heart is at least 20-fold lower (0.1 fmole/mg membrane protein). Therefore, while the beneficial effect of certain GHS-R ligands on cardiac function is a consistent finding, recent studies indicate that a receptor other than the GHS-R is involved. The scavenger receptor CD36 was identified following crosslinking of a ^{125}I-hexarelin analog to heart membranes and the functional significance of this observation was shown by the loss of hexarelin-mediated cardioprotection in CD36 knockout mice (Bodart et al. 1999; Ong et al., Serono Conference on GH in Aging, Florida, October 2001).

GHS-R competition binding studies and ligand activation of site-directed mutants of the GHS-R have been completed. Binding studies show that adenosine acts through a different site than GHRP-6, MK-0677 and ghrelin. Ligand activation of GHS-R mutants demonstrates that ghrelin acts through a distinct but overlapping site than that of GHRP-6 and MK-0677. For example, mutation of E124 in the third transmembrane helix to Q124 produces a receptor that is activated by ghrelin but not by GHRP-6 or MK-0677. Similarly, an analogue of the human GHS-R that we cloned from the Pufferfish can be activated by both GHRP-6 and MK-0677. Hence, the GHS-R has been conserved for at least 400 million years of evolution (Palyha et al. 2000). Surprisingly, ghrelin does not activate the Pufferfish receptor and peptides made by simple modifications of ghrelin by deacylation or amidation of the C-terminus are also inactive on the Pufferfish GHS-R. We are currently using human/Pufferfish GHS-R chimeras to identify the ghrelin activation domain.

The evidence is compelling from *in vitro* studies that ghrelin is a ligand for the GHS-R. Ghrelin and MK-0677 have the same affinity for the GHS-R. In vivo, like the synthetic ligands, ghrelin stimulates feeding behavior and GH release (Asakawa et al. 2001; Cummings et al. 2001; Kamegai et al. 2001; Lawrence et al. 2002; Shintani et al. 2001; Tschop et al. 2001; Wren et al. 2000, 2001a, b). However, it is not yet clear that the GHS-R is the physiologically relevant receptor for ghrelin. If we assume that ghrelin is 100 % bioavailable for binding to its receptor and all the peptide is octanoylated, the concentration measured in serum appears too low (< 1 pM) to be a physiological activator of GH release. The Kd of ghrelin for GHS-R = 1 nM. Unlike ghrelin, MK-0677 does not stimulate gut motility, and chronically, MK-0677 does not result in fat deposition (Masuda et al. 2000; Ravussin et al. 2001; Tschop et al. 2000, 2002). Computer modeling of synthetic GHS-R ligands, ghrelin and truncated ghrelins fail to produce close matches.

An important question to be addressed is how are the different metabolic effects of ghrelin and MK-0677 reconciled. An obvious possibility is that a different GHS-R subtype is activated by ghrelin. The *GHS-R* consists of two exons and encodes two products, 1a and 1b (Howard et al. 1996). The former is a typical, seven-transmembrane (7TM) spanning G-protein coupled receptor, whereas 1b contains TM1-5, which is encoded by exon-1, but lacks TM6 and TM7, which are encoded by exon-2., Using RNAase protection assays, we first demonstrated that GHS-R 1a is expressed almost exclusively in the brain and anterior pituitary gland (Guan et al. 1997; Smith et al. 1999). Although subsequent reports using RT-PCR claim that GHS-R is expressed in a variety of peripheral tissues, in all but one of these studies, the PCR primers fail to discriminate 1a from 1b. Another possibility is that the GHS-R is not the physiologically important receptor for ghrelin and that the ghrelin receptor is the product of another gene. However, after an exhaustive search, we have been unable to identify a candidate with homology to the GHS-R (Smith et al. 2001).

Metabolic Set point

Increases in appetite and fat deposition have been observed in rodents following ghrelin treatment (Tschop et al. 2000; Wren et al. 2001b). These effects are accompanied by increased corticosterone and therefore might be mediated indirectly by glucocorticoids. However, in obese humans chronically treated with MK-0677 for two months, fat deposition and cortisol levels were unaffected, but lean mass and metabolic rate increased (Svensson et al. 1998). From a metabolic perspective, it is counterintuitive that an orexigenic hormone like ghrelin would both increase fat deposition and GH release. However, perhaps the orexigenic properties of ghrelin are regulated at lower levels than those required for stimulating GH release. Ghrelin, in further contrast to MK-0677, has been reported to stimulate gut motility and have effects on cardiovascular tissue (Nagaya et al. 2001a; Masuda et al. 2000).

One explanation for the contrasting effects of ghrelin and MK-0677 are the presence of GHS-R subtypes. To explain the different activities of ghrelin and the synthetic GHS-R ligands, we have recently established two transgenic mouse lines, in which in one case the *ghrelin* and in the other the *GHS-R* genes have been deleted (manuscripts in preparation). The mice of both lines are viable, of normal size and fertility and appear to be behaviorally normal with normal appetite.

The hormone leptin appears to have a counter-regulatory role to ghrelin by inhibiting feeding behavior. However, in pathological situations ghrelin's relationship with leptin appears paradoxical. In obesity, leptin is elevated and ghrelin is low and in anorexia nervosa the opposite is true (Shintani et al. 2001; Shiiya et al. 2002; Wren et al. 2001a; Otto et al. 2001). One explanation that could readily be tested is that, through the hypothalamic/pituitary axis, ghrelin and leptin operate as a metabolic switch. For example, when body fat and hence leptin are low, ghrelin stimulates both feeding and deposition of fat until a specific "set point" is reached. At this set point leptin produced by fat acts in concert with ghrelin on GHS-Rs on arcuate neurons and pituitary somatotrophs to induce release of GHRH and GH. The combined effects of ghrelin and leptin increase GH and IGF-1 levels to balance the distribution of fat and lean tissue.

Conclusion

It is clear that ghrelin and leptin play an important role in regulating feeding behavior through their actions in the hypothalamus. It is uncertain whether they control metabolism and whether their activities are interdependent. A complicating factor is that ghrelin and the longer acting GHS-R ligands produce different biological responses, suggesting that ghrelin is acting on more than one GHS-R subtype. Therefore, we await the results of studies in *ghrelin –/–* and *GHS-R –/–* mice, which provide the tools necessary to facilitate our understanding of the interplay between ghrelin and leptin in the control of metabolism.

References

Asakawa A, Inui A, Kaga T, Yuzuriha H, Nagata T, Ueno N, Makino S, Fujimiya M, Niijima A, Fujino MA, Kasuga M (2001) Ghrelin is an appetite-stimulatory signal from stomach with structural resemblance to motilin. Gastroenterology 120: 337–345

Barzilai N, Gupta G (1999) Interaction between aging and syndrome X: new insights on the pathophysiology of fat distribution. Ann NY Acad Sci 892: 58–72

Bernardis LL, Davis PJ (1996) Aging and the hypothalamus: research perspectives. Physiol Behav 59: 523–536

Bodart V, Bouchard JF, McNicoll N, Escher E, Carriere P, Ghigo E, Sejlitz T, Sirois MG, Lamontagne D, Ong H (1999) Identification and characterization of a new growth hormone-releasing peptide receptor in the heart. Circ Res 85: 796–802

Bowers CY (1996) Xenobiotic growth hormone secretagogues: growth hormone releasing peptides. In: Bercu BB, Walker RF (eds.) Growth hormone secretagogues. Springer-Verlag, New York, pp 9–28

Bowers CY, Momany FA, Reynolds GA, Hong A (1984) On the *in vitro* and *in vivo* activity of a new synthetic hexapeptide that acts on the pituitary to specifically release growth hormone. Endocrinology 114: 1537–1545

Bowers CY, Reynolds GA, Durham D, Barrera CM, Pezzoli SS, Thorner MO (1990) Growth hormone (GH)-releasing peptide stimulates GH release in normal man and acts synergistically with GH-releasing hormone. J Clin Endocrinol Metab 70: 975–982

Chapman IM, Bach MA, Van C, E, Farmer M, Krupa DA, Taylor AM, Schilling LM, Cole KY, Skiles EH, Pezzoli SS, Hartman ML, Veldhuis JD, Gormley GJ, Thorner MO (1996a) Stimulation of the growth hormone (GH)-insulin-like growth factor-I axis by daily oral administration of a GH secretagogue (MK-0677) in healthy elderly subjects. J Clin Endocrinol Metab 81: 4249–4257

Chapman IM, Hartman ML, Pezzoli SS, Thorner MO (1996b) Enhancement of pulsatile growth hormone secretion by continuous infusion of a growth hormone-releasing peptide mimetic, L-692,429, in older adults – a clinical research center study. J Clin Endocrinol Metab 81: 2874–2880

Chapman IM, Pescovitz OH, Murphy G, Treep T, Cerchio CA, Krupa D, Gertz B, Polvino WJ, Skiles EH, Pezzoli SS, Thorner MO (1997) Oral administration of growth hormone (GH) releasing peptide-mimetic MK-677 stimulates the GH/IGF-1 axis in selected GH-deficient adults. J Clin Endocrinol Metab 82: 3455–3463

Cheng K, Chan WW-S, Butler BS, Barreto A, Smith RG (1989) The synergistic effects of His-D-Trp-Ala-Trp-D-Phe-Lys-NH2 on GRF stimulated growth hormone release and intracellular cAMP accumulation in rat primary pituitary cell cultures. Endocrinology 124: 2791–2797

Cheng K, Chan WW-S, Butler BS, Barreto A, Smith RG (1991) Evidence for a role of protein kinase-C in His-D-Trp-Ala-Trp-D-Phe-Lys-NH2-induced growth hormone release from rat primary pituitary cells. Endocrinology 129: 3337–3342

Chihara K, Kashio Y, Kita T, Okimura Y, Kaji H, Abe H, Fujita T (1986) L-dopa stimulates release of hypothalamic growth hormone-releasing hormone in humans. J Clin Endocrinol Metab 62: 466–473

Cincotta AH, Schiller BC, Landry RJ, Herbert SJ, Miers WR, Meier AH (1993) Circadian neuroendocrine role in age-related changes in body fat stores and insulin sensitivity of the male Sprague-Dawley rat. Chronobiol Int 10: 244–258

Colao A, Cuocolo A, Di Somma C, Cerbone G, Della Morte AM, Nicolai E, Lucci R, Salvatore M, Lombardi G (1999) Impaired cardiac performance in elderly patients with growth hormone deficiency. J Clin Endocrinol Metab 84: 3950–3955

Cummings DE, Purnell JQ, Frayo RS, Schmidova K, Wisse BE, Weigle DS (2001) A preprandial rise in plasma ghrelin levels suggests a role in meal initiation in humans. Diabetes 50: 1714–1719

Davey HW, McLachlan MJ, Wilkins RJ, Hilton DJ, Adams TE (1999) STAT5b mediates the GH-induced expression of SOCS-2 and SOCS-3 mRNA in the liver. Mol Cell Endocrinol 158: 111–116

Dean DC, Nargund RP, Pong S-S, Chaung L-YP, Griffin PR, Melillo DG, Ellsworth RL, Van der Ploeg LHT, Patchett AA, Smith RG (1996) Development of a high specific activity sulfur-35-labeled sulfonamide radioligand that allowed the identification of a new growth hormone secretagogue receptor. J Med Chem 39: 1767–1770

De Gennaro Colonna V, Rossoni G, Bernareggi M, Muller EE, Berti F (1997a) Cardiac ischemia and impairment of vascular endothelium function in hearts from growth hormone-deficient rats: protection by hexarelin. Eur J Pharmacol 334: 201–207

De Gennaro Colonna V, Rossoni G, Bernareggi M, Muller EE, Berti F (1997b) Hexarelin, a growth hormone-releasing peptide, discloses protectant activity against cardiovascular damage in rats with isolated growth hormone deficiency. Cardiologia 42: 1165–1172

Ferre S, Fredholm BB, Morelli M, Popoli P, Fuxe K (1997) Adenosine-dopamine receptor-receptor interactions as an integrative mechanism in the basal ganglia. TINS 20: 482–487

Fletcher TP, Thomas GB, Clarke IJ (1996) Growth hormone-releasing hormone and somastatin concentrations in the hypophysial portal blood of conscious sheep during the infusion of growth hormone-releasing peptide-6. Domestic Animal Endocrinol 13: 251–258

Guan XM, Yu H, Palyha OC, McKee KK, Feighner SD, Sirinathsinghji DJ, Smith RG, Van der Ploeg LH, Howard AD (1997) Distribution of mRNA encoding the growth hormone secretagogue receptor in brain and peripheral tissues. Brain Res Mol Brain Res 48: 23–29

Guillaume V, Magnan E, Cataldi M, Dutour A, Sauze N, Renard M, Razafindraibe H, Conte-Devolx B, Deghenghi R, Lenaerts V, Oliver C (1994) Growth hormone (GH)-releasing hormone secretion is stimulated by a new GH-releasing hexapeptide in sheep. Endocrinology 135: 1073–1076

Hewson AK, Dickson SL (2000) Systemic administration of ghrelin induces Fos and Egr-1 proteins in the hypothalamic arcuate nucleus of fasted and fed rats. J Neuroendocrinol 12: 1047–1049

Ho KY, Evans WS, Blizzard RM, Veldhuis JD, Merriam GR, Samojlik E, Furlanetto R, Rogol AD, Kaiser DL, Thorner MO (1987) Effects of sex and age on the 24-hour profile of growth hormone secretion in man: importance of endogenous estradiol concentrations. J Clin Endocrinol Metab 64: 51–58

Hoffman GE, Sladek JR, Jr. (1980) Age-related changes in dopamine, LHRH and somatostatin in the rat hypothalamus. Neurobiol Aging 1: 27–37

Howard AD, Feighner SD, Cully DF, Arena JP, Liberator PA, Rosenblum CI, Hamelin M, Hreniuk DL, Palyha OC, Anderson J, Paress PS, Diaz C, Chou M, Liu KK, McKee KK, Pong S-S, Chaung L-YP, Elbrecht A, Dashkevicz M, Heavens R, Rigby M, Sirinathsinghji DJS, Dean DC, Melillo DG, Patchett AA, Nargund RP, Griffin PR, DeMartino JA, Gupta SK, Schaeffer JM, Smith RG, Van der Ploeg LHT (1996) A receptor in pituitary and hypothalamus that functions in growth hormone release. Science 273: 974–977

Jansson JO, Eden S, Isaksson O (1985) Sexual dimorphism in the control of growth hormone secretion. Endocr Rev 6: 128–150

Kamegai J, Tamura H, Shimizu T, Ishii S, Sugihara H, Wakabayashi I (2001) Chronic central infusion of ghrelin increases hypothalamic neuropeptide Y and Agouti-related protein mRNA levels and body weight in rats. Diabetes 50: 2438–2443

Katugampola SD, Pallikaros Z, Davenport AP (2001) [125I-His(9)]-ghrelin, a novel radioligand for localizing GHS orphan receptors in human and rat tissue: up-regulation of receptors with atherosclerosis. Brit J Pharmacol 134: 143–149

Kish SJ, Shannak K, Rajput A, Deck JH, Hornykiewicz O (1992) Aging produces a specific pattern of striatal dopamine loss: implications for the etiology of idiopathic Parkinson's disease. J Neurochem 58: 642–648

Kojima M, Hosoda H, Date Y, Nakazato M, Matsuo H, Kangawa K (1999) Ghrelin is a growth-hormone-releasing acylated peptide from stomach. Nature 402: 656–660

Lawrence CB, Snape AC, Baudoin FM, Luckman SM (2002) Acute central ghrelin and GH secretagogues induce feeding and activate brain appetite centers. Endocrinology 143: 155–162

Masuda Y, Tanaka T, Inomata N, Ohnuma N, Tanaka S, Itoh Z, Hosoda H, Kojima M, Kangawa K (2000) Ghrelin stimulates gastric acid secretion and motility in rats. Biochem Biophys Res Commun 276: 905–908

Matsumoto AM, Marck BT, Gruenewald DA, Wolden-Hanson T, Naai MA (2000) Aging and the neuroendocrine regulation of reproduction and body weight. Exp Gerontol 35: 1251–1265

Miller JD, Tannenbaum GS, Cole E, Guyda HJ (1982) Daytime pulsatile growth hormone secretion during childhood and adolescence. J. Clin. Endocrinol. Metab. 55: 989–994

Momany FA, Bowers CY, Reynolds GA, Chang D, Hong A, Newlander K (1981) Design, synthesis, and biological activity of peptides which release growth hormone, in vitro. Endocrinology 108: 31–39

Murphy MG, Plunkett LM, Gertz BJ, He W, Wittreich J, Polvino WM, Clemmons DR (1998) MK-0677, an orally active growth hormone secretagogue reverses diet-induced catabolism. J Clin Endocrinol Metab 83: 320–325

Murphy MG, Bach MA, Plotkin D, Bolognese J, Ng J, Krupa D, Cerchio K, Gertz BJ (1999) Oral administration of the growth hormone secretagogue MK-677 increases markers of bone turnover in healthy and functionally impaired elderly adults. The MK-677 Study Group. J Bone Miner Res 14: 1182–1188

Nagaya N, Miyatake K, Uematsu M, Oya H, Shimizu W, Hosoda H, Kojima M, Nakanishi N, Mori H, Kangawa K (2001a) Hemodynamic, renal, and hormonal effects of ghrelin infusion in patients with chronic heart failure. J Clin Endocrinol Metab 86: 5854–5859

Nagaya N, Uematsu M, Kojima M, Ikeda Y, Yoshihara F, Shimizu W, Hosoda H, Hirota Y, Ishida H, Mori H, Kangawa K (2001b) Chronic administration of ghrelin improves left ventricular dysfunction and attenuates development of cardiac cachexia in rats with heart failure. Circulation 104: 1430–1435

Ongini E, Fredholm BB (1996) Pharmacology of adenosine A_{2A} receptors. Trends Pharmacol. Sci. 17: 364–372

Otto B, Cuntz U, Fruehauf E, Wawarta R, Folwaczny C, Riepl RL, Heiman ML, Lehnert P, Fichter M, Tschop M (2001) Weight gain decreases elevated plasma ghrelin concentrations of patients with anorexia nervosa. Eur J Endocrinol 145: 669–673

Palyha OC, Feighner SD, Tan CP, McKee KK, Hreniuk DL, Gao Y-D, Schleim KD, Yang L, Morriello GJ, Nargund R, Patchett AA, Howard AD, Smith RG (2000) Ligand activation domain of human orphan growth hormone secretagogue receptor (GHS-R) conserved from Pufferfish to humans. Mol. Endocrinol. 14: 160–169

Patchett AA, Nargund RP, Tata JR, Chen M-H, Barakat KJ, Johnston DBR, Cheng K, Chan WW-S, Butler BS, Hickey GJ, Jacks TM, Scleim K, Pong S-S, Chaung L-YP, Chen HY, Frazier E, Leung KH, Chui S-HL, Smith RG (1995) The design and biological activities of L–163,191 (MK–0677): a potent orally active growth hormone secretagogue. Proc Natl Acad Sci USA 92: 7001–7005

Pong S-S, Chaung L-Y, Dean DC, Nargund RP, Patchett AA, Smith RG (1996) Identification of a new G-protein-linked receptor for growth hormone secretagogues. Mol Endocrinol 10: 57–61

Porter JC, Kedzierski W, Aguila-Mansilla N, Jorquera BA (1990) Expression of tyrosine hydroxylase in cultured brain cells: stimulation with an extractable pituitary cytotropic factor. Endocrinology 126: 2474–2481

Porter JC, Aguila-Mansilla N, Ramin SM, Kozlowski GP, Kedzierski W (1991) Tyrosine hydroxylase expression in hypothalamic cells: analysis of the roles of adenosine 3',5'-monophosphate- and Ca2+/calmodulin-dependent protein kinases in the action of pituritary cytotropic factor. Endocrinology 129: 2477–2485

Porter JC, Ijames CF, Wang T-CL, Markey SP (1995) Purification and identification of pituitary cytotropic factor. Proc Natl Acad Sci USA 92: 5351–5355

Premont J, Perez M, Bockaert J (1977) Adenosine-sensitive adenylate cyclase in rat striatal homogenates and its relationship to dopamine- and Ca^{2+}-sensitive adenylate. Mol Pharmacol 13: 662–670

Ram PA, Park SH, Choi HK, Waxman DJ (1996) Growth hormone activation of Stat 1, Stat 3, and Stat 5 in rat liver. Differential kinetics of hormone desensitization and growth hormone stimulation of both tyrosine phosphorylation and serine/threonine phosphorylation. J Biol Chem 271: 5929–5940

Ravussin E, Tschop M, Morales S, Bouchard C, Heiman ML (2001) Plasma ghrelin concentration and energy balance: overfeeding and negative energy balance studies in twins. J Clin Endocrinol Metab 86: 4547–4551

Rossoni G, Locatelli V, De Gennaro Colonna V, Torsello A, Schweiger F, Boghen M, Nilsson M, Bernareggi M, Muller EE, Berti F (1999) Growth hormone and hexarelin prevent endothelial vasodilator dysfunction in aortic rings of the hypophysectomized rat. J Cardiovasc Pharmacol 34: 454–460

Rudman D, Feller AG, Hoskote S, Nagraj HS, Gergans GA, Lalitha PY, Goldberg AF (1990) Effects of growth hormone in men over 60 years old. N Engl J Med 323: 1–6

Satinoff E, Li H, Tcheng TK, Liu C, McArthur AJ, Medanic M, Gillette MU (1993) Do the suprachiasmatic nuclei oscillate in old rats as they do in young ones? Am J Physiol 265: R1216–1222

Scarpace PJ, Matheny M, Moore RL, Tumer N (2000) Impaired leptin responsiveness in aged rats. Diabetes 49: 431–435

Shiiya T, Nakazato M, Mizuta M, Date Y, Mondal MS, Tanaka M, Nozoe S, Hosoda H, Kangawa K, Matsukura S (2002) Plasma ghrelin levels in lean and obese humans and the effect of glucose on ghrelin secretion. J Clin Endocrinol Metab 87: 240–244

Shintani M, Ogawa Y, Ebihara K, Aizawa-Abe M, Miyanaga F, Takaya K, Hayashi T, Inoue G, Hosoda K, Kojima M, Kangawa K, Nakao K (2001) Ghrelin, an endogenous growth hormone secretagogue, is a novel orexigenic peptide that antagonizes leptin action through the activation of hypothalamic neuropeptide Y/Y1 receptor pathway. Diabetes 50: 227–232

Smith RG, Cheng K, Schoen WR, Pong S-S, Hickey GJ, Jacks TM, Butler BS, Chan WW-S, Chaung L-YP, Judith F, Taylor AM, Wyvratt MJ, Jr., Fisher MH (1993) A nonpeptidyl growth hormone secretagogue. Science 260: 1640–1643

Smith RG, Cheng K, Pong S-S, Leonard RJ, Cohen CJ, Arena JP, Hickey GJ, Chang CH, Jacks TM, Drisko JE, Robinson ICAF, Dickson SL, Leng G (1996a) Mechanism of action of GHRP-6 and nonpeptidyl growth hormone secretagogues. In: Bercu BB, Walker RF (eds) Growth hormone secretagogues. Serono Symposia. Springer-Verlag, New York, pp 147–163

Smith RG, Pong S-S, Hickey GJ, Jacks TM, Cheng K, Leonard RJ, Cohen CJ, Arena JP, Chang CH, Drisko JE, Wyvratt MJ, Jr., Fisher MH, Nargund RP, Patchett AA (1996b) Modulation of pulsatile GH release through a novel receptor in hypothalamus and pituitary gland. Rec. Prog Horm Res 51: 261–286

Smith RG, Van der Ploeg LH, Howard AD, Feighner SD, Cheng K, Hickey GJ, Wyvratt MJ, Jr., Fisher MH, Nargund RP, Patchett AA (1997) Peptidomimetic regulation of growth hormone secretion. Endocr Rev 18: 621–645

Smith RG, Feighner S, Prendergast K, Guan X, Howard A (1999) A new orphan receptor involved in pulsatile growth hormone release. Trends Endocrinol. Metab. 10: 128–135

Smith RG, Griffin PR, Xu Y, Smith AG, Liu K, Calacay J, Feighner SD, Pong C, Leong D, Pomes A, Cheng K, Van der Ploeg LH, Howard AD, Schaeffer J, Leonard RJ (2000) Adenosine: A partial agonist of the growth hormone secretagogue receptor. Biochem Biophys Res Commun 276: 1306–1313

Smith RG, Leonard R, Bailey AR, Palyha O, Feighner S, Tan C, McKee KK, Pong SS, Griffin P, Howard A (2001) Growth hormone secretagogue receptor family members and ligands. Endocrine 14: 9–14

Sonntag WE, Forman LJ, Miki N, Trapp JM, Gottschall PE, Meites J (1982) L-dopa restores amplitude of growth hormone pulses in old male rats to that observed in young male rats. Neuroendocrinology 34: 163–168

Steiner RA, Stewart JK, Barber J, Koerker D, Gooner CJ, Brown A, Illner P, Gale CC (1978) Somatostatin: a physiological role in the regulation of growth hormone secretion in the adolescent male baboon. Endocrinology 102: 1587–1594

Svensson J, Lonn L, Jansson J-O, Murphy G, Wyss D, Krupa D, Cerchio K, Polvino W, Gertz B, Boseaus I, Sjostrom L, Bengtsson B-A (1998) Two-month treatment of obese subjects with the oral growth hormone (GH) secretagogue MK-677 increases GH secretion, fat-free mass, and energy expenditure. J Clin Endocrinol Metab 83: 362–369

ThyagaRajan S, MohanKumar PS, Quadri SK (1995) Cyclic changes in the release of norepinephrine and dopamine in the medial basal hypothalamus: effects of aging. Brain Res 689: 122–128

Tivesten A, Bollano E, Caidahl K, Kujacic V, Sun XY, Hedner T, Hjalmarson A, Bengtsson BA, Isgaard J (2000) The growth hormone secretagogue hexarelin improves cardiac function in rats after experimental myocardial infarction. Endocrinology 141: 60–66

Tschop M, Smiley DL, Heiman ML (2000) Ghrelin induces adiposity in rodents. Nature 407: 908–913

Tschop M, Wawarta R, Riepl RL, Friedrich S, Bidlingmaier M, Landgraf R, Folwaczny C (2001) Post-prandial decrease of circulating human ghrelin levels. J Endocrinol Invest 24: RC19–21

Tschop M, Statnick MA, Suter TM, Heiman ML (2002) GH-releasing eptide-2 increases fat mass in mice lacking NPY: indication for a crucial mediating role of hypothalamic Agouti-related protein. Endocrinology 143: 558–568

Tullin S, Hansen BS, Ankersen M, Moller J, Von Cappelen KA, Thim L (2000) Adenosine is an agonist of the growth hormone secretagogue receptor. Endocrinology 141: 3397–3402

Wang ZW, Pan WT, Lee Y, Kakuma T, Zhou YT, Unger RH (2001) The role of leptin resistance in the lipid abnormalities of aging. Faseb J 15: 108–114

Wren AM, Seal LJ, Cohen MA, Brynes AE, Frost GS, Murphy KG, Dhillo WS, Ghatei MA, Bloom SR (2001a) Ghrelin enhances appetite and increases food intake in humans. J Clin Endocrinol Metab 86: 5992.

Wren AM, Small CJ, Abbott CR, Dhillo WS, Seal LJ, Cohen MA, Batterham RL, Taheri S, Stanley SA, Ghatei MA, Bloom SR (2001b) Ghrelin causes hyperphagia and obesity in rats. Diabetes 50: 2540–2547

Wren AM, Small CJ, Ward HL, Murphy KG, Dakin CL, Taheri S, Kennedy AR, Roberts GH, Morgan DG, Ghatei MA, Bloom SR (2000) The novel hypothalamic peptide ghrelin stimulates food intake and growth hormone secretion. Endocrinology 141: 4325–4328

Yamagami K, Joseph JA, Roth GS (1992) Muscarinic receptor concentrations and dopamine release in aged rat striata. Neurobiol Aging 13: 51–56

Yurek DM, Hipkens SB, Hebert MA, Gash DM, Gerhardt GA (1998) Age-related decline in striatal dopamine release and motoric function in brown Norway/Fischer 344 hybrid rats. Brain Res 791: 246–256

Regulation of Galanin-Like Peptide (GALP) in the Brain and Posterior Pituitary: A Review

A. Juréus[1], D. K. Clifton[2] and R. A. Steiner[1,2,3]

Summary

Galanin-like peptide (GALP) is a recently discovered neuropeptide. GALP shares a partial sequence homology with galanin, and it binds and activates several galanin receptor subtypes. In the brain, the distribution of GALP-containing cell bodies is restricted to the arcuate nucleus (Arc), median eminence (ME) and infundibular stalk (IS) of the medial basal hypothalamus. In the Arc, GALP neurons express the signaling form of the leptin receptor (Ob-Rb). Levels of GALP mRNA in the Arc are reduced with fasting and induced by leptin, reminiscent of leptin's effect on the expression of proopiomelanocortin and cocaine-amphetamine regulated transcript. GALP neurons in the Arc send efferent projections to areas in the rostral hypothalamus, where they appear in close proximity to gonadotropin-releasing hormone (GnRH) cell bodies and fibers. When GALP is delivered into the brain, it stimulates the release of LH through a GnRH-dependent mechanism. GALP is also expressed in pituicytes in the neuronal lobe of the pituitary, and its expression there is induced by dehydration and salt-loading. The purpose of this review is to summarize the existing knowledge about GALP, discuss its possible physiological significance and provide a perspective for future investigations.

Introduction

Galanin is a neuropeptide, which that expressed abundantly in many regions of the brain and periphery and has been implicated in numerous physiological processes (Bartfai et al. 1993; Merchenthaler et al. 1993; Kask et al. 1997). For example, galanin-producing cells are present in several hypothalamic nuclei concerned with the control of pituitary function and the regulation of metabolism (Melander et al. 1986). Galanin is co-expressed in a subset of gonadotropin-releasing hormone (GnRH) neurons in the medial preoptic area (MPOA) and is believed to play a role in reproduction and sexual behavior (Merchenthaler et al. 1990; Merchenthaler 1991; Hohmann et al. 1998; Finn et al. 1996). Galanin is also co-expressed with growth hormone (GH)-releasing hormone (GHRH) in the arcuate nucleus, and in this context, galanin is thought to participate in the regula-

Departments of [1]Physiology & Biophysics, [2]Obstetrics & Gynecology and [3]Zoology, University of Washington, Seattle, WA 98195-7290, USA

Kordon et al.
Brain Somatic Cross-Talk and the
Central Control of Metabolism
© Springer-Verlag Berlin Heidelberg 2002

tion of GH secretion (Delemarre -van de Weal et al. 1994). Galanin is expressed in a subpopulation of lactotropes in the anterior pituitary (Hsu et al. 1990), is co-localized with oxytocin and vasopressin in magnucellular neurons of the paraventricular nucleus (PVN), and is thought to play a crucial role during lactation in the female rat (Wynick et al. 1993a, 1998; Landry et al. 1991, 1997; Eriksson et al. 1996). Furthermore, several lines of evidence suggest that galanin is an important signal in the control of food intake and regulation of body weight, having primarily orexigenic properties (Crawley 1999; Leibowitz 1994). Outside the hypothalamus, galanin plays a role in higher cognitive function, including learning and memory, and is associated with certain neurological disorders, including epilepsy, depression, and Alzheimer's and Parkinson's diseases (Chan-Palay 1988; Steiner et al. 2001; Mufson et al. 1998; Crawley 1996; Weiss et al. 1998; Mazarati et al. 2000). In the spinal cord, galanin is present in the dorsal root ganglion, where it is thought to be involved in the modulation of sensory processing and pain (Xu et al. 2000; Wiesenfeld-Hallin and Xu 1998; Wiesenfeld-Hallin et al. 1992).

Galanin mediates its actions through G-protein coupled receptors, of which three different subtypes (GalR1-GalR3) have been cloned and found to be expressed in the hypothalamus(Branchek et al. 2000). These three receptors have different distributions and activate different signal transduction pathways. GalR1 and GalR3 appear to have a preference for Gi/Go proteins inhibiting andenylate cyclase and opening K^+ channels, and thus have a hyperpolarizing effect (Habert-Ortoli et al. 1994; Parker et al. 1995; Smith et al. 1998). GalR2 activates Gq/G11-like proteins to stimulate phospholipase C and releases Ca^{2+} from intracellular stores (Smith et al. 1997; Wang et al. 1998; Fathi et al. 1998). Galanin binds to all three of galanin's known receptors (GalR1-3) with high affinity. The first 13 amino acids of galanin (counted from the N-terminus) are highly conserved among species. This part of the molecule also comprises the biological activity of the peptide, and galanin 1-13 by itself acts as a full agonist (Bartfai et al. 1992). The distribution of GalR1 and GalR2 mRNA in the brain has been characterized in the rat by in situ hybridization and overlaps well with the distribution of galanin-binding sites. GalR1 is widely expressed throughout the hypothalamus, with robustly labeled cells being evident in dorsomedial nucleus (DMN), ventromedial nucleus (VMN), and PVN, and with lower levels of expression evident in almost all other hypothalamic nuclei. Within the hypothalamus, the distribution of GalR2 is more restricted than that of GalR1. In the hypothalamus, the highest levels of GalR2 mRNA are found in the mammillary body and Arc (O'Donnel et al. 1999; Waters and Krause 2000; Mitchell et al. 1999; Depczynski et al. 1998; Landry et al. 1999; Gustafson et al. 1996), and notably, GalR2 (but not GalR1 or 3) is expressed in the anterior pituitary (Depczynski et al. 1998).

The discovery of GALP

Until December 1999, galanin was structurally unrelated to any known regulatory peptide or family of peptides in the mammalian brain – notwithstanding the suggestion by several groups that other unknown galanin-like peptides in all likelihood exist. The cross-reactivity of galanin antiserum and discrepancies in the pharmacology of chimeric galanin receptor ligands, which antagonize galanin in vivo and act as agonists at the three cloned galanin receptors in vitro, implied the existence of an additional endogenous ligand for these receptors that should be structural by related to galanin (Smith et al. 1997, 1998; Wang et al. 1997; Rökaeus et al. 1984).

Recently, Ohtaki and his colleagues isolated a novel galanin-like peptide (GALP) from the porcine hypothalamus by seeking galanin-like activity, as reflected by [^{35}S]GTPγS binding to cell membranes from CHO cell transfected with galanin receptors (Ohtaki et al. 1999). GALP was identified as a 60 amino acid peptide, which unlike galanin has a non-amidated C-terminus. Curiously, 13 amino acid residues of the GALP sequence (9–21) were completely identical to the highly conserved N-terminal 13 residues of galanin (Ohtaki et al. 1999). These 13 residues comprise the primary site of interaction with the known galanin receptor subtypes and are necessary for high affinity binding. The same 13 amino acids are also the core sequence for the design of chimeric galanin receptor ligands (Langel and Bartfai 1998). To date, GALP has been cloned from five different species – are rat, pig, human, mouse and monkey – and the 13 residues showing identity to galanin are 100 % conserved among all these species (Ohtaki et al. 1999; Juréus et al. 2001; Cunningham et al. 2002). Pharmacological evaluation of synthetic GALP revealed that GALP recognizes both GalR1 (IC50=4.3 nM) and GalR2 (IC50=0.24 nM) with high affinity, but with an 18-fold preference to the GalR2 receptor subtype (Ohtaki et al. 1999). Agonistic activity of GALP has been established through the use of a [^{35}S]GTPγS binding assay. Potent agonistic activity was obtained for both GalR1 and GalR2, with a 180-fold greater agonist activity at GalR2 compared to GalR1, suggesting that GALP is more selective for GalR2 (Ohtaki et al. 1999). GALP's pharmacology at GalR3 has not yet been investigated. Recently, the GALP gene was localized to chromosome 19 in the human and mapped to reveal six putative exons (Cunningham et al. 2002).

Distribution of GALP mRNA expressing cells in the brain and pituitary

Shortly after the discovery of the GALP peptide and the cloning of GALP cDNAs, the distribution of GALP mRNA in the rat brain and pituitary was investigated by in situ hybridization (Juréus et al. 2000; Larm and Gundlach 2000; Kerr et al. 2000; Takatsu et al. 2001). These investigations revealed that in the brain GALP mRNA-expressing cells have a remarkably restricted distribution in all species examined to date, in contrast to galanin. In the brain of the rat, GALP mRNA-containing cells are found only in the Arc, ME, and IS of the hypothalamus. GALP mRNA-expressing cells are also observed in the neural lobe, notably in pituicytes, which are a type of glial cell (Juréus et al. 2000; Shen et al. 2001). No GALP-expressing cells could be detected in the hippocampus, thalamus, amygdala, or brain stem, areas that express high levels of galanin receptors. Likewise, no GALP-expressing cells could be identified in dorsal root ganglion, which is also known to express high levels of both GalR1 and GalR2 (Kerr et al. 2000). Within the Arc, the anatomical localization of GALP cells has a very distinct and unique pattern. The majority of GALP cells are found in the caudal part of the Arc, with a high number of cells appearing in the very medial aspect surrounding the third ventricle. A similar periventricular expression pattern is observed in the mouse, although in this species, GALP cells are found more laterally and appear to be distributed more uniformly throughout the full rostral-caudal extent of the nucleus (Juréus et al. 2001). In the monkey, the expression of GALP mRNA approximates that of the rat and mouse (Cunningham et al. 2002). The pattern of GALP expression in the Arc is different from that of galanin, which is distributed more laterally in the nucleus. Although there may be some modest overlap, the general anatomical distribution of GALP mRNA-expressing cells in the Arc is distinct from that of any other commonly recognized peptide in the Arc, such as neuropeptide Y (NPY), galanin, proopiomelanocortin (POMC), GHRH, cocaine and amphetamine-regulated transcript (CART), agouti-related protein (AGRP) and somatostatin. Furthermore, none of the cells containing any of these neuropeptides would appear to co-express GALP, at least not in the rat (Takatsu et al. 2001). The finding of GALP-containing cells in the ME and IS is particularly intriguing, since this circumventricular area contains relatively few neurons, arguing that these GALP-containing cells may be some other cell type, such glia. The restricted expression of GALP cells in the medial basal hypothalamus and posterior pituitary suggests that GALP may serve a neuroendocrine or neurosecretory function.

Projections of GALP-containing neurons

Using monoclonal antibodies directed towards the N-terminal sequence GALP (1–10), Takatsu and his colleagues (2001) mapped the distribution of GALP immunoreactivity in the brain of the rat. GALP immuno-positive cell bodies were found exclusively in the Arc, ME and IS, corroborating the earlier reported distribution of cells expressing GALP mRNA (Juréus et al. 2000; Larm and Gundlach 2000; Kerr et al. 2000; Takatsu et al. 2001). GALP-containing fibers were observed in several brain regions, including the PVN, the bed nucleus of the stria terminalis (BST), the lateral septum (LS), the hypothalamic periventricular nucleus (PeN), and the medial preoptic area (MPOA). Notably, no GALP fibers were observed in the external zone of the ME, suggesting that GALP cells in the Arc do not project to the hypophysial portal system. Thus, GALP would seem unlikely to serve as a hypophysiotropic hormone. Within the PVN, GALP-containing fibers are found in the anterior parvocellular part of the PVN. This distribution is notably different from galanin- and AGRP-containing fibers, which are distributed mainly in the medial part of the PVN and only occasionally in the parvicellular part of the nucleus (Takatsu et al. 2001). These fiber projections most likely originate from the Arc, since it is the only brain region known to express GALP mRNA (Fig. 1).

GALP is regulated by leptin in the Arc

Leptin is a hormone secreted by adipocytes and acts on the brain to regulate appetite, metabolism, and pituitary function (Friedman and Halaas 1998; Friedman

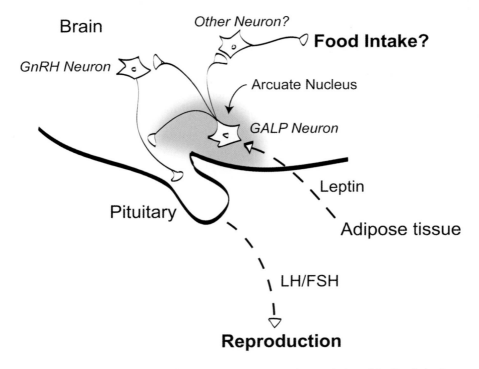

Fig. 1. Schematic drawing illustrating the role of GALP in the regulation of feeding behaviour and the neuroendocrine reproductive axis. GALP neurons in the arcuate nucleus are stimulated by leptin. GALP synthesis and secretion are induced, which signals (+) to GnRH neurons in the MPOA and BST. The release of GnRH stimulates the secretion of LH and FSH from the pituitary. GALP also acts on other peptidergic neurons in the hypothalamus to inhibit feeding. The effect of leptin on GALP gene expression is reminiscent of ist stimulatory effect on other anorectic neuropeptides in the arcuate nucleus, such als α-MSH and CART, suggesting that GALP acts along with these and other peptides to regulate feeding and metabolism, as well as reproduction.

2000). Leptin acts on the signaling form of the homodimeric leptin receptor, Ob-Rb, to transduce its effects in the hypothalamus (Tartaglia et al. 1995). Ob-Rb is highly expressed in the Arc, where leptin is known to regulate the transcription of leptin-responsive pepdidergic neurons such as orexigenic NPY/AGRP neurons and anorectic POMC/CART neurons (Thornton et al. 1997; Kristensen et al. 1998; Schwartz et al. 1996; Ollmann et al. 1997). Noting that the expression of GALP is limited to the Arc and that its distribution overlaps with Ob-Rb, we surmised that GALP might be a target for regulation by leptin. To test this hypothesis, we measured levels of GALP mRNA in three experimental groups of female rats. Two groups were fasted (representing a state of low leptin levels) for 48 hours and they received (sc) injections of either leptin (5 ug/g body wt) or vehicle solution, twice daily. The third group was allowed to feed ad libitum and injected with vehicle

(Juréus et al. 2000). Fasting reduced the number of GALP mRNA-containing cells by half in the Arc, whereas treatment with leptin reversed the fasting-induced inhibition of GALP expression and increased the number of detectable GALP cells in the Arc four-fold over that of the fasted/vehicle-treated group. Leptin's stimulatory effect on GALP mRNA was further corroborated by studies in the leptin-deficient ob/ob mouse (Juréus et al. 2001). There were far fewer identifiable GALP neurons in the Arc of the ob/ob mouse compared to wild-type controls. Moreover, this phenotype could be fully reversed by central (icv) infusions of leptin, arguing persuasively that GALP neurons in the Arc are responsive to leptin. This conclusion is further strengthened by the finding that a large fraction (88 %) of GALP-immunopositive cells in the Arc of the rat also stain positively for leptin receptor (OB-R; Takatsu et al. 2001). A similar co-localization study in the monkey has also confirmed that nearly all of the GALP mRNA-expressing cells co-express Ob-Rb mRNA (Cunningham et al. 2002). The effect of leptin on the regulation of GALP gene-expression is reminiscent of its stimulatory effect on anorectic POMC/CART neurons in the Arc, suggesting GALP may serve as a mediator of leptin's effect on feeding, metabolism, and possibly reproduction.

GALP stimulates luteinizing hormone (LH) secretion in the male rat

Takatsu and colleagues found that GALP neurons send projections to the forebrain including the PVN, MPOA, BST and the LS (Takatsu et al. 2001). Using double-label immunostaining, they also discovered that GALP-containing fibers are in close approximation to GnRH perikarya in the ventrolateral part of the MPOA and also appear in close association with GnRH fibers in the MPOA and BST. These findings suggest that there may be functional interaction between GnRH and GALP neurons in the regulation of the neuroendocrine reproductive axis. This is consistent with leptin's putative role in the regulation of reproductive function (Cunningham et al. 1999). Shortly thereafter, it was demonstrated that central (icv) administration of GALP to male rats (5 nmol/rat) caused a significant increase in plasma LH levels compared to vehicle-treated animals, peaking 30 minutes after administration (Matsumoto et al. 2001). Pretreating rats with a GnRH receptor antagonist blocks this activity, arguing that the action of GALP on LH secretion was mediated by GnRH. The same dose of centrally infused galanin failed to generate any response on LH secretion, suggesting that the effect of GALP on LH secretion may have been mediated by a unique GALP receptor (unrecognized by galanin). Furthermore, icv injections of GALP induced the expression of the intermediate early gene c-fos in GnRH neurons, adding credibility to the notion that GALP induces transcriptional activity in GnRH neurons. On the other hand, GALP had no effect on the basal release of LH from dispersed anterior pituitary cells, suggesting that GALP does not have a direct effect on the gonadotropes of the anterior pituitary. These elegant studies demonstrate that GALP could mediate the effects of leptin on GnRH secretion and thus serve as a molecular motif linking body weight regulation and reproduction.

Functional significance of GALP in the posterior pituitary, IS and ME

GALP mRNA-expressing cells are present in the IS, ME and posterior pituitary – areas that contain relatively few neuronal perikarya. In the adult rat, the majority of the GALP mRNA-expressing cells in the posterior pituitary are found in its inner region. Using combined in situ hybridization and immunohistochemistry, Shen and colleagues demonstrated that GALP mRNA is expressed in cells also staining for glial fibrillary acidic protein (GFAP), a glial marker, suggesting GALP is synthesized in the pituicytes of the posterior pituitary (Shen et al. 2001). The neurosecretory activity of vasopressinergic (AVP or antidiuretic hormone, ADH) neurons is highly sensitive to changes in plasma osmolality, and these cells are stimulated by dehydration and salt-loading. Terminals of magnocellular neurons containing AVP and oxytocin, originating from the PVN and supraoptic nucleus (SON), are localized to the posterior pituitary, and the levels of both of these peptides are altered by osomotic challenge (Falke 1991). Shen and co-workers performed a study in rats measuring GALP gene expression in the posterior pituitary following water deprivation and salt-loading. After this osmotic challenge, there was a dramatic (~40-fold) increase in the expression of GALP mRNA in the posterior pituitary compared to controls. In addition, the area of the posterior pituitary shown to contain cells that express GALP mRNA was increased to cover both the inner *and* outer regions of the neurohypophysis. This observation suggests that GALP may play a role in the secretory activity of the posterior pituitary and could thus serve an important function in the regulation of fluid balance, lactation and perhaps the morphological organization of the neurohypophysis itself. Although the presence and regulation of GALP would imply that it has some physiological significance in the control of posterior pituitary function, its cousin galanin is notably absent from the posterior lobe.

Concluding remarks

The discovery of GALP has added a new and fascinating dimension to research on the galanin family of peptides. GALP shares a partial sequence identity with galanin in a stretch of 13 highly conserved amino acids, which comprise all of the major pharmacophores of galanin (Ohtaki et al. 1999). In vitro GALP is able to recognize and activate both GalR1 and GalR2, with a preference for the GalR2 subtype. However, GALP's ability to bind and stimulate the third of the known galanin receptors (GalR3) has not yet been investigated. Pharmacological evidence suggests the presence of additional galanin receptor subtypes (Wynick et al. 1993b; Hedlund et al. 1992; Rossowski et al. 1190; Xu et al. 1999), and there is a distinct possibility that one or more unique receptors exist for GALP itself. The C-terminus of GALP (22-60) has no sequence homology with galanin, yet it contains segments of amino acids sequences that are highly conserved among species. This observation marks this region of the GALP molecule as a possible site for interaction with one or more possible GALP-specific receptors. Further investigations mapping GALP binding sites and GALP-induced activities in the brain, which are unique from those of galanin, are necessary steps towards elucidating the pharmacology of GALP, as well as its close cousin, galanin.

GALP-expressing neurons in the hypothalamus are localized exclusively in the Arc (Juréus et al. 2000; Larm and Gundlach 2000; Kerr et al. 2000), which is a nodal point for the control of important neuroendocrine functions, such as the regulation of feeding, metabolism and pituitary hormone secretion. Many neurons whose cell bodies reside in the Arc are responsive to leptin. These cells express neuropeptides, such as NPY/AGRP (orexigenic) and CART/POMC (anorectic), which then signal the presence or absence of leptin to other hypothalamic regions for integration and subsequent modulation of appetitive behaviors, metabolism and reproductive function (Thornton et al. 1997; Kristensen et al. 1998; Schwartz et al. 1996; Ollmann et al. 1997). Leptin stimulates the transcriptional activity of GALP neurons, similar to its effect on POMC/CART neurons in the Arc (Juréus et al. 2000, 2001), suggesting that GALP might act along with POMC-derived peptides and CART to inhibit food intake and stimulate metabolism. Future experiments investigating whether systemically administered leptin activates signaling mechanisms downstream of the leptin receptor, such as c-fos, SOCS-3 and STAT3, will establish whether there is a direct leptin-triggered activation of the full transcriptional machinery present in GALP neurons within the Arc.

Some cells in the Arc, such as POMC neurons, make direct contact with hypohysiotropic neurons in the PVN and MPOA (e.g., GnRH neurons; Cheung and Hammer 1995), and leptin is known to be involved in the regulation of the secretion of several pituitary hormones, including ACTH, TSH, and the gonadotropins (Casanueva and Dieguez 1999). However, the signaling mechanisms that mediate this function are poorly understood. GALP cells in the Arc send projections to brain regions in the forebrain including the PVN, MPOA and BST, and GALP-containing fibers appear in close proximity to GnRH neurons in the MPOA and BST (Takatsu et al. 2001). In addition, when GALP is injected directly into the brain, it can stimulate the release of LH in a GnRH-dependent manner (Matsumoto et al. 2001). Leptin can reverse the delay of puberty caused by mild food restriction and corrects the infertility phenotype of the ob/ob mouse (Cunningham et al. 1999; Clarke and Henry 1999). Taken together, these observations suggest that GALP might be a physiological mediator of leptin's action in the regulation of the neuroendocrine reproductive axis. Additional experiments involving the administration of GALP for longer periods in experimental animals are necessary to validate the significance of GALP's role in the regulation of the reproductive axis.

GALP is also produced by specialized glia cells in the posterior pituitary, where GALP gene expression is induced by dehydration or salt-loading (Shen et al. 2001). These pituicytes are known to control the release of AVP and oxytocin from hypothalamic magnocellular neurons by altering the mechanical and chemical environment around their axon terminals in the posterior pituitary (Falke 1991; Hatton 1990). GALP's proximate localization to these specialized neurosecretory regions of oxytocin and AVP neurons and its transcriptional regulation by osmotic challenge suggest that GALP may play a role in the regulation of fluid balance and possibly lactation.

Many neuropeptides are expressed in both the brain and peripheral organs, where they serve functions distinct from their roles as either neurotransmitters or hypophysiotropic factors in the brain. Galanin receptors are widely expressed throughout the CNS, as well as in many peripheral organs (Branchek et al. 2000); however to date, GALP-expressing cells have not been reported to exist outside the brain and pituitary. Nevertheless, based on this history of neuropeptides, it seems plausible, even likely, that GALP is expressed in other tissues in the periphery, where it may serve as either a hormone or paracrine factor. A thorough screening for GALP expression in peripheral organs might unmask new and important functions for this novel peptide.

In summary, we have just begun to understand the functional significance of GALP. The application of both classical and modern transgenic and antisense strategies coupled with the development of more selective ligands for galanin receptors should provide important clues about the role of GALP in physiology and disease.

References

Bartfai T, Fisone G, Langel Ü (1992) Galanin and galanin antagonists: molecular and biochemical perspectives. Trends Pharmacol Sci 13:312–317

Bartfai T, Hökfelt T, Langel Ü (1993) Galanin – a neuroendocrine peptide. Crit Rev Neurobiol 7:229–274

Branchek TA, Smith KE, Gerald C, Walker MW (2000) Galanin receptor subtypes. Trends Pharmacol Sci 21:109–117

Casanueva FF, Dieguez C (1999) Neuroendocrine regulation and actions of leptin. Front Neuroendocrinol 20:317-363

Chan-Palay V (1988) Neurons with galanin innervate cholinergic cells in the human basal forebrain and galanin and acetylcholine coexist. Brain Res Bull 21:465–472

Cheung S, Hammer RP (1995) Gonadal steroid hormone regulation of proopiomelanocortin gene expression in arcuate neurons that innervate the medial preoptic area of the rat. Neuroendocrinology 62:283–292

Clarke IJ, Henry BA (1999) Leptin and reproduction. Rev Reprod 4:48–55

Crawley JN (1996) Minireview. Galanin-acetylcholine interactions: relevance to memory and Alzheimer's disease. Life Sci 58:2185–2199

Crawley JN (1999) The role of galanin in feeding behavior. Neuropeptides 33:369–375

Cunningham MJ, Clifton DK, Steiner RA (1999) Leptin's actions on the reproductive axis: perspectives and mechanisms. Biol Reprod 60:216–222

Cunningham MJ, Scarlett JM, Clifton DK, Steiner RA (2002) Cloning and distribution of galanin-like peptide (GALP) mRNA in the brain and pituitary of the macaque. Endocrinology, in press

Delemarre-van de Waal HA, Burton KA, Kabigting EB, Steiner RA, Clifton DK (1994) Expression and sexual dimorphism of galanin messenger ribonucleic acid in growth hormone-releasing

Depczynski B, Nichol K, Fathi Z, Iismaa T, Shine J, Cunningham A (1998) Distribution and characterization of the cell types expressing GALR2 mRNA in brain and pituitary gland. Ann NY Acad Sci 863:120–128

Eriksson M, Ceccatelli S, Uvnäs-Moberg K, Iadaroly M, Hökfelt T (1996) Expression of Fos-related antigens, oxytocin, dynorphin and galanin in the paraventricular and supraoptic nuclei of lactating rats. Neuroendocrinology 63:356–367

Falke N (1991) Modulation of oxytocin and vasopressin release at the level of the neurohypophysis. Prog Neurobiol 36:465–484

Fathi Z, Cunningham AM, Iben LG, Battaglino PB, Ward SA, Nichols KA, Pine KA, Wang J, Goldstein ME, Ismaa TP, Zimayi IA (1998) Cloning, pharmacological characterizatioin and distribution of a novel galanin receptor. Brain Res Mol Brain Res 53:348

Finn PD, McFall TB, Clifton DK, Steiner RA (1996) Sexual differentiation of galanin gene expression in gonadotropin-releasing hormone neurons. Endocrinology 137:4767–4772

Friedman JM (2000) Obesity in the new mellenium. Nature 404:632–634

Friedman JM, Halaas J (1998) Leptin and the regulation of body weight in mammals. Nature 395:763–770

Gustafson EL, Smith KE, Durkin MM, Gerald C, Branchek TA (1996) Distribution of a rat galanin receptor mRNA in rat brain. Neuroreport 7:953–957

Habert-Ortoli E, Amiranoff B, Loquet I, Laburthc M, Mayaux JF (1994) Molecular cloning of a functional human galanin receptor. Proc Natl Acad Sci USA 91:9780–9783

Hatton GI (1990) Emerging concepts of structure-function dynamics in adult brain: The hypothalamo-neurohypophysial system. Prog Neurobiol 34:437–504

Hedlund PB, Yanaihara N, Fuxe K (1992) Evidence for specific N-terminal galanin fragment binding sites in the rat brain. Eur J Pharmacol 224:203–205

Hohmann JG, Clifton DK, Steiner RA (1998) Galanin: analysis of its coexpression in gonadotropin-releasing hormone and growth hormone-releasing hormone neurons. Ann NY Acad Sci 863:221–235

hormone neurons of the rat during development. Endocrinology 134:665–671

Hsu DW, el-Azouzi M, Black PM, Chin WW, Hedley-Whyte ET, Kaplan LM (1990) Estrogen increases galanin immunoreactivity in hyperplastic prolactin-secreting cells in Fisher 344 rats. Endocrinology 126:3159–3167

Juréus A, Cunningham MJ, Li D Johnson LL, Krasnow SM, Teklemichael DN, Clifton DK, Steiner RA (2001) Distribution and regulation of galanin-like peptide (GALP) in the hypothalamus of the mouse. Endocrinology 142:5140–5144

Juréus A, Cunningham MJ, Mcclain ME, Clifton DK, Steiner RA (2000) Galanin-like peptide (GALP) is a target for regulation by Leptin in the hypothalamus of the rat. Endocrinology 141:2703–2706

Kask K, Berthold M, Bartfai T (1999) Galanin receptors: involvement in feeding, pain, depression and Alzheimer's disease. Life Sci 60:1523–1533

Kerr NC, Holmes FE, Wynick D (2000) Galanin-like peptide (GALP) is expressed in rat hypothalamus and pituitary, but not in DRG. Neuroreport 11:3909–3913

Kristensen P, Judge ME, Thim L, Ribel U, Christjansen KN, Wulff BS, Clausen JT, Jens PB, Madsen OD, Vrang N, Lawen PJ, Hastup S (1998) Hypothalamic CART is a new anorectic peptide regulated by leptin. Nature 393:72–76

Landry M, Aman K, Burlet A, Hökfelt T (1999) Galanin-R1 receptor mRNA expression in the hypothalamus of the Brattelboro rat. Neuroreport.10:2823–2827

Landry M, Roche D, Angelova E, Calas A (1997) Expression of galanin in hypothalamic magnocellular neurones of lactating rats: co-existence with vasopressin and oxytocin. J Endocrinol 155:467–481

Landry M, Trembleau A, Arai R, Calas A (1991) Evidence for a colocalization of oxytocin mRNA and galanin in magnocellular hypothalamic neurons: a study combining in situ hybridization and immunohistochemistry. Brain Res Mol Brain Res 10:91–95

Langel Ü, Bartfai T (1998) Chemistry and molecular biology of galanin receptor ligands. Ann NY Acad Sci 863:86–93

Larm JA, Gundlach AL (2000) Galanin-like peptide (GALP) mRNA expression is restricted to arcuate nucleus of hypothalamus in adult male rat brain. Neuroendocrinology 72:67–71

Leibowitz SF (1994) Specificity of hypothalamic peptides in the control of behavioral and physiological processes. Ann NY Acad Sci 739:12–35

Matsumoto H, Noguchi J, Takatsu Y, Horikoshi Y, Kumano S, Ohtaki T, Kitada C, Itoh T, Onda H, Nishimuna O, Fujino M (2001) Stimulation of galanin-like peptide (GALP) on lutenizing hormone-releasing hormone-mediated lutenizing hormone (LH) secretion in male rats. Endocrinology 142:3693–3696

Mazarati AM, Hohmann JG, Bacon A, Liu H, Sankar R, Steiner RA, Wynick D, Wasterlain CG (2000) Modulation of hippocampal excitability and seizures by galanin. J Neurosci 20:6276–6281

Melander T, Hökfelt T, Rokaeus A (1996) Distribution of galaninlike immunoreactivity in the rat central nervous system. J Comp Neurol 248:475–517

Merchenthaler I (1991) The hypophysiotropic galanin system of the rat brain. Neuroscience 44:643–654

Merchenthaler I, Lopez FJ, Negro-Vilar A (1990) Colocalization of galanin and luteinizing hormone-releasing hormone in a subset of preoptic hypothalamic neurons: anatomical and functional correlates. Proc Natl Acad Sci USA 87:6326–6330

Merchenthaler I, Lopez FJ, Negro-Vilar A (1999) Anatomy and physiology of central galanin-containing pathways. Prog Neurobiol 40:711–769

Mitchell V, Bouret S, Howard AD, Beauvillain JC (1999) Expression of the galanin receptor subtype Gal-R2 mRNA in the rat hypothalamus. J Chem Neuroanat 16:265–277

Mufson EJ, Kahl U, Bowser R, Mash DC, Kordower JH, Deecher DC (1998) Galanin expression within the basal forebrain in Alzheimer's disease. Comments on therapeutic potential. Ann NY Acad Sci 863:291–304

O'Donnell D, Ahmad S, Wahlestedt C, Walker P (1999) Expression of the novel galanin receptor subtype GALR2 in the adult rat CNS: distinct distribution from GALR1. J Comp Neurol 409:469–481

Ohtaki T, Kumano S, Ishibashi Y, Ogi K, Matsui H, Harada M, Kitada C, Kurokawa T, Onda H, Fujino M (1999) Isolation and cDNA cloning of a novel galanin-like peptide (GALP) from porcine hypothalamus. J. Biol. Chem. 274:37041–37045

Ollmann M, Wilson BD, Yang Y-K, Kerns JA, Chen Y, Gantz I, Baush GS (1997) Antagonism of central melanocortin receptors in vitro and in vivo by agouti-related protein. Science 278:135–138

Parker EM, Izzarelli DG, Nowak HP, Mahle CD, Iben LG, Wang J, Goldstein ME (1995) Cloning and characterization of the rat GALR1 galanin receptor from Rin14B insulinoma cells. Brain Res Mol Brain Res 4:179–189

Rökaeus A, Melander T, Hökfelt T, Lundberg JM, Tatemoto K, Calquist M, Mutt V (1984) A galanin-like peptide in the central nervous system and intestine of the rat. Neurosci Lett 47:161–166

Rossowski WJ, Rossowski TM, Zacharia S, Ertan A, Coy DH (1990) Galanin binding sites in rat gastric and jejunal smooth muscle membrane preparations. Peptides 11:333–338

Schwartz MV, Baskin DG, Bukowsky TR, Kuipen JL, Forster D, Lasser G, Prunkard DE, Ponte DJR, Woods SC, Seeley RJ, Weigle DS (1996) Specificity of leptin action on elevated blood glucose levels and hypothalamic neuropeptide Y gene expression in *ob/ob* mice. Diabetes 45:531–535

Shen J, Larm J, Gundlach AL (2001) Galanin-like peptide mRNA in the neural lobe of rat pituitary. Increased expression after osmotic stimulation suggests a role for galanin-like peptide in neuronal-glial interactions and/or neurosecretion. Neuroendocrinology 73:2–11

Smith KE, Forray C, Walker MW, et al. (1997) Expression cloning of a rat hypothalamic galanin receptor coupled to phosphoinositide turnover. J Biol Chem 272:24612–24616

Smith KE, Walker MW, Artymyshyn R, Bard J, Borowsky B, Tamm JA, Yao WS, Vaysse PSS, Branchek TA, Gerald C, Jones KA (1998) Cloned human and rat galanin GALR3 receptors. Pharmacology and activation of G-protein inwardly rectifying K+ channels. J Biol Chem 273:23321–23326

Steiner R, Hohmann J, Holmes A, Wrenn CC, Cadd G, Junéus A, Clifton DK, Luo M, Gutschall M, Ma SY, Mufson EJ, Crawley JN (2001) Galanin transgenic mice display cognitive and neuro-chemical deficits characteristic of Alzheimer's disease. Proc Natl Acad Sci USA 98:4184–4189

Takatsu Y, Matsumoto H, Ohtaki T, Kumano S, Kitada C, Onda H, Nishimura O, Fujino M (2001) Distribution of galanin-like peptide in the brain. Endocrinology 142:1626–1634

Tartaglia LA, Dembski M, Wenig X, Deng N, Culpeper J, Devos R, Richards GJ, Campfield LA, Clark FT, Deeds J (1995) identification and coling of a leptin receptor OB-R. Cell 83:1263–1271

Thronton JE, Cheung CC, Clifton DK, Steiner RA (1997) Regulation of hypothalamic proopi-omelanocortin mRNA by leptin in *ob/ob* mice. Endocrinology 138:5063–5066

Wang S, Hashemi T, Fried S, Clemmons AL, Hawes BE (1998) Differential intracellular signaling of the Ga1R1 and Ga1R2 galanin receptor subtypes. Biochemistry 37:6711–6717

Wang ZL, Kulkarni RN, Wang RM, Smith DM, Ghatei MA, Byfield PG, Bennet WM, Bloom SR (1997) Possible evidence for endogenous production of a novel galanin-like peptide. J Clin invest 100:189–196

Waters SM, Krause JE (2000) Distribution of galanin-1, -2, and -3 receptor messenger RNAs in central and peripheral rat tissues. Neuroscience 95:265–271

Weiss JM, Bonsall RW, Demetrikopoulos MK, Emery MS, West CH (1998) Galanin: a significant role in depression? Ann NY Acad Sci 863:364–382

Wiesenfeld-Hallin Z, Bartfai T, Hökfelt T (1992) Galanin in sensory neurons in the spinal cord. Front Neuroendocrinol 13:319–343

Wiesenfeld-Hallin Z, Xu XJ (1998) Galanin in somatosensory function. Ann NY Acad Sci 863:383–389

Wynick D, Hammond PJ, Akinsanya KO, Bloom SR (1993a) Galanin regulates basal and oestro-gen stimulated lactotroph function. Nature 364:529–532

Wynick D, Small CJ, Bacon A, Holmes FE, Noreman M, Oremandy CJ, Kilic E, Kerr NCH, Ghatei M, Takamantes F, Bloom SR, Pachuis V. (1998) Galanin regulates prolactin release and lac-totroph proliferation. Proc Natl Acad Sci USA 95:12671–12676

Wynick D, Smith DM, Ghatei M, Akinsaya K, Bhogal R, Purkiss P, Byfield P, Yancihara N, Bloom SR (1993b) Characterization of a high-affinity galanin receptor in the rat anterior pituitary: absence of biological effect and reduced membrane binding of the antagonist M15 differen-tiate it from the brain/gut receptor. Proc Natl Acad Sci USA 90:4231–4235

Xu XJ, Hökfelt T, Bartfai T, Wiesenfeld-Hallin Z (2000) Galanin and spinal nociceptive mecha-nisms: recent advances and therapeutic implications. Neuropeptides 34:137–147

Xu Z-QD, Ma X, Soomets U, Langel G, Hökfelt T (1999) Electrophysiological evidence for a hyperpolarizing galanin (1-15)-selective receptor on hippocampal CA3 pyramidal neurons. Proc Nat Acad Sci USA 96:14583–14587

Ghrelin and the Growth Hormone Neuroendocrine Axis

G. S. Tannenbaum[1], J. Epelbaum[2], and C. Y. Bowers[3]

Summary

Growth hormone (GH) is an anabolic hormone that is essential for normal linear growth and has important metabolic effects throughout life. The ultradian rhythm of GH secretion is generated by the intricate patterned release of two hypothalamic hormones, somatostatin (SRIF) and GH-releasing hormone (GHRH), acting both at the level of the pituitary gland and within the central nervous system. The recent discovery of ghrelin, a novel GH-releasing peptide identified as the endogenous ligand for the GH-secretagogue receptor (GHS-R) and shown to induce a positive energy balance, suggests the existence of an additional neuroendocrine pathway for GH control. To further understand how ghrelin interacts with the classical GHRH/SRIF neuronal system in GH regulation, we used a combined physiological and histochemical approach. Our physiologic studies of the effects of ghrelin on spontaneous pulsatile GH secretion in conscious, free-moving rats demonstrate that: 1) ghrelin, administered peripherally, exerts potent, time-dependent GH-releasing activity under physiological conditions; 2) ghrelin is a functional antagonist of SRIF, but its GH-releasing activity is not dependent on inhibiting endogenous SRIF release; 3) SRIF antagonizes the action of ghrelin acting at the level of the pituitary gland; and 4) the GH response to ghrelin requires an intact endogenous GHRH system. Our dual chromogenic and autoradiographic in situ hybridization experiments provide anatomical evidence that ghrelin may directly modulate GHRH mRNA- and NPY mRNA-containing neurons in the hypothalamic arcuate nucleus, but that SRIF mRNA-expressing cells in the periventricular nucleus are not major direct targets for ghrelin. Together, these findings support the notion that ghrelin may be a critical hormonal signal of nutritional status to the GH neuroendocrine axis serving to integrate energy balance and the growth process.

[1]Departments of Pediatrics and of Neurology and Neurosurgery, McGill University, and the Neuropeptide Physiology Laboratory, McGill University-Montreal Children's Hospital Research Institute, Montreal, Québec H3H 1P3, Canada
[2]Institut National de la Santé et de la Recherche Médicale U549, 75014 Paris, France
[3]Department of Medicine, Division of Endocrinology, Tulane University Medical Center, New Orleans, Louisiana 70112–2699, USA

Kordon et al.
Brain Somatic Cross-Talk and the
Central Control of Metabolism
© Springer-Verlag Berlin Heidelberg 2002

Introduction

Growth hormone (GH) is an anabolic hormone that is essential for normal linear growth. In addition, GH has important metabolic effects on a variety of physiological systems throughout life. These non-growth effects include facilitating the utilization of fat mass for energy stores, building and sustaining lean body mass, and maintaining bone mineral density (Carrel and Allen 2000).

Regulation of the secretion of GH from the anterior pituitary gland is under the control of at least two hypothalamic hormones, a stimulatory GH-releasing hormone (GHRH) found in the arcuate nucleus, and an inhibitory hormone, somatostatin (SRIF), synthesized in the periventricular nucleus. Several lines of evidence suggest that, in addition to the intricate patterned release of GHRH and SRIF regulating GH directly at the pituitary level, SRIF modulates GH secretion indirectly through central regulation of GHRH-containing neurons. The net result of these interactions is a striking pulsatile pattern of GH release as observed in the peripheral blood of both human and experimental animals (see Fig 1; also Tannenbaum and Epelbaum 1999 for review).

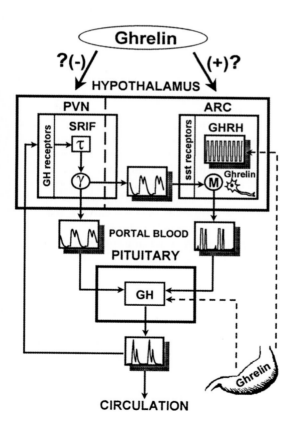

Fig. 1. Schematic drawing of the signaling pathway of the GH neuroendocrine axis for generation of the ultradian rhythm of GH secretion in the rat. SRIF and GHRH are released from the hypothalamus into the portal blood at approximately 3.3 h intervals. At the pituitary, the reciprocal release patterns of GHRH and SRIF result in a GH profile in the circulation as shown. SRIF is also rhythmically secreted within the hypothalamus at the level of the arcuate nucleus (ARC), where it affects GHRH neurons (for further description of the model see Wagner et al. 1998). To what degree stomach ghrelin versus hypothalamic ghrelin, or both, plays a physiological role in the control of pulsatile GH secretion at the level of either the pituitary or brain remains to be determined. PNV: paraventricular nucleus.

In recent years, there has been intense interest in a novel class of peptide and non-peptidyl synthetic compounds, termed GH secretagogues (GHSs), developed from the prototype hexapeptide GHRP-6 (Bower et al. 1984) and shown to exert potent GH-releasing activity in multiple species, including humans (Smith et al. 1997; Bowers 1999). A unique receptor for GHS (GHS-R) was cloned from the pituitary of humans (Howard et al. 1996) and rats (McKee et al. 1997), and numerous sites of expression of GHS-R were identified the brain (Guan et al. 1997). Double-labeling studies demonstrated the expression of GHS-R by GHRH mRNA-containing neurons in the hypothalamus (Tannenbaum et al 1998a; Willesen et al. 1999), suggesting that GHSs might directly modulate GHRH neurons. Moreover, GHS-R mRNA, in both brain (Bennett et al. 1997)) and pituitary (Kamegai et al. 1998), was shown to be sensitive to changes in GH status. All these findings supported the notion that a third neuroendocrine pathway may exist to regulate pulsatile GH secretion.

The breakthrough discovery, in late 1999, of the natural endogenous ligand for the GHS-R, termed ghrelin (Kojima et al. 1999), has provided a new and intriguing dimension for GH research. The chemistry and the major anatomical site of origin of ghrelin are novel; it is a Ser^3-octanoylated 28 amino acid peptide that surprisingly originates primarily from the stomach rather than the hypothalamus, although ghrelin-immunoreactive neurons have been detected in small amounts in the hypothalamic arcuate nucleus in rats (Kojima et al. 1999; Lu et al. 2002) and humans (Korbonits et al. 2001). Ghrelin is a potent GH secretagogue, both in vitro and in vivo, in rats and humans (Kojima et al. 1999; Seoane et al. 2000; Takaya et al,. 2000; Arvat et al. 2000). However, the neuroendocrine pathways through which ghrelin acts to release GH relative to the classical hypothalamic regulators of GH secretion, and its functional significance for GH regulation, are largely unknown (Fig. 1).

Intriguingly, ghrelin's actions are not restricted to the GH axis. Ghrelin also functions as a powerful orexigenic hormone; it stimulates feeding and increases body weight when administered either peripherally or centrally (Tschöp et al. 2000; Nakazato et al. 2001; Wren et al. 2000), and these effects appear to be independent of changes in GH (Tschöp et al. 2000; Nakazato et al. 2001). It is well known that the secretion of GH is exquisitely sensitive to perturbations in nutritional status (see Tannenbaum and Epelbaum 1999 for review); thus ghrelin may be a critical hormonal signal of nutritional status to the GH neuroendocrine axis.

In this paper, we report on our physiological studies designed to further understand how ghrelin interacts with the well-established, seemingly self-sufficient GHRH/SRIF neuronal system in regulation of GH secretion. To determine the hypothalamic cell types through which ghrelin influences GH release and food intake, we performed dual chromogenic and autoradiographic in situ hybridization and examined/compared the co-expression of the GHS-R with SRIF, GHRH and Neuropeptide Y (NPY), neuropeptides involved in GH regulation and feeding behavior.

Materials and Methods

Animals and experimental procedures

Adult male Sprague-Dawley rats (225–300 g) were purchased from Charles River Canada (St. Constant, Canada) and individually housed on a 12-h light, 12-h dark cycle (lights on, 0600–1800 h) in a temperature- (22 ± 1 C)- and humidity-controlled room. Purina rat chow (Ralston Purina, St. Louis, MO) and tap water were available ad libitum.

For the physiological studies, chronic intracardiac venous cannulae were implanted under sodium pentobarbitol (50 mg/kg, ip) anesthesia using a previously described technique (Tannenbaum and Martin 1976). After surgery, the rats were placed directly in isolation test chambers with food and H_2O freely available until body weight returned to preoperative levels (usually within five to seven days). On the test day, food was removed 1.5 h before the start of sampling and was returned at the end.

In the first series of experiments, we examined the temporal pattern and magnitude of the GH response to ghrelin. Free-moving rats were given iv injections of either 5 µg ghrelin or normal saline at two different time points during a six-hour sampling period. The times of 1100 and 1300 h were chosen since these times reflect typical peak and trough periods of GH secretion, as previously documented (Tannenbaum and Martin 1976; Tannenbaum and Ling 1984)). The human ghrelin peptide (kindly provided by Dr. K. Chang, Phoenix Pharmaceuticals, Belmont, CA) was diluted in normal saline just before use. Blood samples (0.35 ml) were withdrawn every 15 min over the six-hour sampling period (1000–1600 h) from all animals. To document the rapidity of the GH response to ghrelin, an additional blood sample was obtained five min after each injection of the peptide. All blood samples were immediately centrifuged, and the plasma was separated and stored at –20 C for subsequent assay of GH. To avoid hemodynamic disturbance, the red blood cells were resuspended in normal saline and returned to the animal after removal of the next blood sample.

In the second series of experiments, designed to assess the roles of endogenous GHRH and SRIF in mediating the GH responses to ghrelin, two groups of rats were administered 1–2 ml of specific GHRH or SRIF antisera iv, at 1000 h, after removal of the first blood sample. The ghrelin peptide (5 µg) was subsequently injected iv at 1100 and 1300 h. A third group of rats served as controls and received 1–2 ml normal sheep serum and 5 µg ghrelin iv at the same time points. Blood samples were withdrawn from 1000–1600 h, as described above. The SRIF and GHRH antisera were the same as those described in our previous passive immunization studies (Tannenbaum and Ling 1984; Painson and Tannenbaum 1991).

For the histochemical studies, adult male Sprague-Dawley rats were killed by decapitation between 1100 and 1115 h. The brains were snap-frozen in isopentane at –40 °C for 1 min and stored at –80 °C. They were coronally sectioned with a cryostat (Leica CM 3050 S), at 20-µm thickness, beginning at the joining of the anterior commissure and continuing caudally to the mammillary bodies. Sections were collected on poly-L-lysine (50 µg/ml)-coated slides, dried for 2 min at 37 °C, and stored at –70 C until in situ hybridization was performed.

All animal-based procedures were approved by the McGill University Animal Care Committee.

GH assay

Plasma GH concentrations were measured in duplicate by double antibody RIA using materials supplied by the NIDDK Hormone Distribution Program (Bethesda, MD). The averaged plasma GH values are reported in terms of the rat GH reference preparation (rGH RP-2). The standard curve was linear between 0.62 and 320 ng/ml; the least detectable concentration of plasma GH under the conditions used was 1.2 ng/ml. All samples with values above 320 ng/ml were reassayed at dilutions ranging from 1:2 to 1:10. The intra- and inter-assay coefficients of variation were 7.7 % and 10.7 %, respectively, for duplicate samples of pooled plasma containing a mean GH concentration of 60.7 ng/ml.

Probe preparation

GHS-R: Single-stranded sense and antisense RNA probes were generated from constructed full-length rat GHS-R type 1a cDNA (a gift from Dr. Andrew Howard, Merck Research Laboratories, Rahway, NJ) inserted into the mammalian expression vector pcDNA3 (Invitrogen Corp., Carlsbad, CA). To obtain GHS-R antisense probes, the cDNA templates were produced by linearization of the vector with *Eco*RI and transcription with the Gemini II system (Promega Biotec, Madison, WI) using SP6 RNA polymerase and [^{35}S]-uridine 5'-[α-thio]triphosphate (DuPont-New England Nuclear, Boston, MA). Sense probes were prepared from *Not*1-linearized plasmid DNA in the presence of T7 RNA polymerase. Aliquots were stored at −70 °C. Before use, the identity and integrity of the probes were verified by PAGE against known standards. The final probe-specific activity was approximately 1.6×10^9 dpm/µg.

GHRH: The rat prghrf-2 plasmid was obtained from Dr. Kelly Mayo, Northwestern University, Evanston, IL. A 217-bp fragment including the entire GHRH-43 coding sequence was subcloned into the transcription vector pGEM-4 (Promega Biotec, Madison, WI), and a digoxigenin (DIG)-labeled antisense cRNA probe was made in vitro using the DIG RNA Labeling Mix (Boehringer Mannheim, Laval, Quebec) containing 3.5 mM DIG-II-UTP; 6.5 mM unlabeled UTP; 10 mM GTP, ATP and CTP; and T7 RNA polymerase.

SRIF and NPY: The rat pSRIF-28 and rat pBLNPY-1 plasmids were obtained from Dr. Robert Steiner, University of Washington School of Medicine, Seattle, WA. DIG-labeled antisense cRNA probes were made in vitro using the DIG RNA Labeling Mix described above, and SP6 RNA polymerase (SRIF probe) or T3 RNA polymerase (NPY probe).

Double label in situ hybridization

We performed dual chromogenic and autoradiographic in situ hybridization using a protocol described previously (Tannenbaum et al. 1998a,b). Separate experiments were carried out for each of the DIG-labeled probes. Briefly, processed sections were hybridized with ^{35}S-labeled antisense GHS-R probe (3–6 $\times$ 10^6 cpm/ml) and either 3.75 µl/ml (GHRH), 2.5 µl/ml (SRIF), or 5 µl/ml (NPY) DIG-labeled antisense probes in hybridization buffer. Overnight hybridization at 60 °C was followed by RNase treatment, a series of stringent SSC washes, and a wash at 60 °C. The slides were then blocked with 2 % normal sheep serum, and incubated overnight at RT with 150 µl of anti-DIG antibody conjugated to alkaline phosphatase (Boehringer Mannheim; 1:1000). Slides were rinsed in buffer before applying 150 µl of chromogen and incubated at 37 °C for seven h until color development. They were then washed in TE, dehydrated in 70 % ethanol, air-dried, dipped in 3 % parlodion and dried overnight. All slides were coated with NTB2 photographic emulsion (Eastman Kodak, Rochester, NY) diluted 1:1 with distilled H_2O and exposed for five to six weeks at 4 °C.

Image analysis

Light microscopic autoradiograms of hybridized brain sections were analyzed under epifluorescence illumination using a computer-assisted image analysis system (Biocom, Les Ulis, France) coupled to a Leitz Diaplan microscope (Leitz, Rockleigh, NJ). Twenty tissue sections per rat for each probe were analyzed. First, the number of GHS-R, GHRH, SRIF and NPY-labeled cells were quantified using Histo and Rag programs; purple-stained DIG-labeled GHRH, SRIF or NPY cells were outlined and counted under brightfield illumination. Second, the number of silver grains overlying individual DIG-labeled cells was counted. Cells were considered double-labeled if the density of silver grains counted over them was at least three times higher than background (determined in another area of the hypothalamus). Results were expressed either as percentage (mean ±SE) of GHRH, SRIF or NPY mRNA-positive cells dually stained for GHS-R mRNA or as percentage of GHS-R mRNA-positive cells expressing GHRH, SRIF, or NPY in the arcuate (ARC), ventromedial (VMN), and periventricular (PeV) nuclei of the hypothalamus.

Statistical analyses

Analysis of variance and Student's t tests for unpaired and paired data, as appropriate, were used for statistical comparisons between and within experimental groups. The results are expressed as the mean ± SE; $P < 0.05$ was considered significant.

Results

Temporal pattern of GH responsiveness to ghrelin

Figure 2 illustrates individual, representative plasma GH responses evoked by ghrelin administered iv during peak and trough periods of GH secretion, compared to normal saline-injected controls. Injection of 5 µg ghrelin during a time of a spontaneous GH secretory episode (1100 h) caused a rapid five- to eight-fold increase in plasma GH levels within five min after injection; plasma GH levels re-

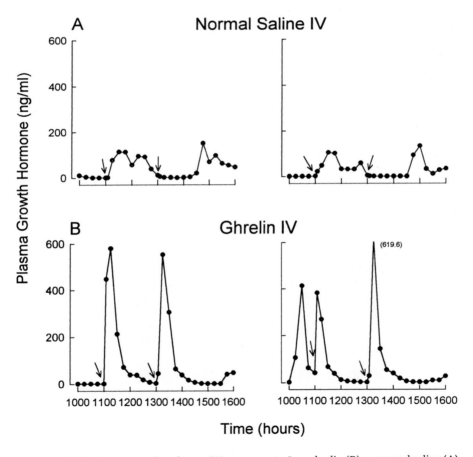

Fig. 2. Individual, representative plasma GH responses to 5 µg ghrelin (**B**) or normal saline (**A**) administered iv during spontaneous peak (1100 h) and trough (1300 h) periods of GH secretion. Ghrelin induced a rapid increase in plasma GH within five min after injection when administered during a spontaneous GH secretory episode; in contrast, the GH response to ghrelin during trough periods was markedly attenuated at five min, with recovery evident only at 15 min. Arrows indicate the times of injections.

mained significantly elevated for approximately 30 min compared to normal, saline-treated controls. In contrast, injection of ghrelin during a trough period (1300 h), when endogenous SRIF release is known to be high (Tannenbaum and Ling 1984), resulted in a markedly attenuated GH response at five min. However, by 15 min, the amount of GH released was similar to that observed at peak times. This time-dependent, GH-releasing activity of ghrelin was also observed at other doses tested; doubling the dose of ghrelin to 10 μg did not significantly alter either the amplitude or temporal pattern of the GH response compared to the 5 μg dose.

Effects of immunoneutralization of endogenous SRIF and GHRH on GH responsiveness to ghrelin

Normal sheep-serum-treated control rats exhibited high ghrelin-induced GH release five min after injection at GH peak times and a minimal five-min response during the GH trough period (Fig. 3). Administration of SRIF antiserum reversed the blunted five-min GH response to ghrelin during trough periods (1300 h) to

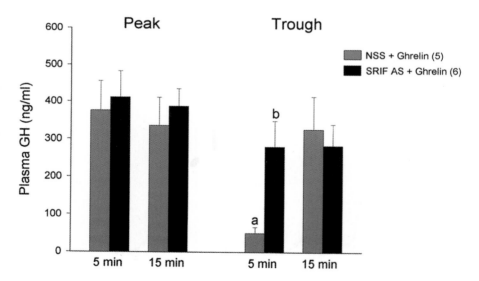

Fig. 3. Effects of passive immunization with SRIF antiserum on mean plasma GH responses to ghrelin (5 μg) administered iv during peak (1100 h) and trough (1300 h) periods of GH secretion. Normal sheep serum (NSS)-treated control rats exhibited high ghrelin-induced GH release five min after injection at peak times and a minimal five-min response at trough times. Administration of SRIF antiserum (SRIF AS) reversed the blunted five-min GH response to ghrelin during trough periods, to levels as high as those observed at peak times. Each bar represents the mean ±SE; the number of animals in each group is shown in *parentheses*. **a.** $P < 0.02$ compared with 5-min GH response to ghrelin at peak times. **b.** $P < 0.01$ compared with NSS-treated controls at the same time point.

levels as high as those observed during peak periods. Of interest, however, is the full recovery of the GH response to ghrelin by 15 min during the trough period, which was consistently observed in all groups (Fig. 3).

In striking contrast, immunoneutralization of endogenous GHRH virtually obliterated the GH responses to 5 μg iv ghrelin observed in normal sheep-serum-treated controls, irrespective of the time administered (Fig. 4).

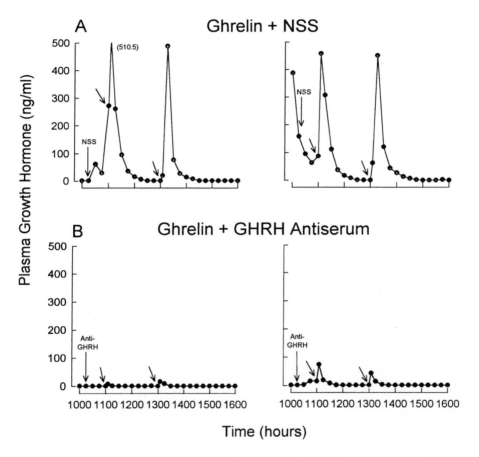

Fig. 4. Effects of GHRH antiserum on GH responsiveness to ghrelin. Immunoneutralization of endogenous GHRH (**B**) virtually obliterated the GH responses to ghrelin (5 μg iv) observed in normal sheep serum (NSS)-treated controls (**A**), irrespective of the time administered. Arrows, times of injections.

Expression of GHS receptors by GHRH, SRIF and NPY neurons

Light microscopic examination of coronal sections taken through the rat brain revealed moderate to strong autoradiographic GHS-R hybridization signal in several hypothalamic and extrahypothalamic regions. Within the hypothalamus, numerous intensely labeled cells were detected throughout the VMN, as well as within the ARC nucleus; more sparsely distributed and/or less intensely labeled neurons were evident in the PeV. SRIF-expressing neurons were also found in these three nuclei but in greater amounts in the PeV. GHRH neurons were only located in the ARC and outer lateral rim of the VMN. NPY expression was restricted to the boundaries of the ARC, in close opposition with the IIIrd ventricle.

At high magnification, there was a clear-cut colocalization of cells located in the zones of the ARC (Fig. 5) and VMN nuclei in which the different populations overlapped. Quantitative analysis of double-labeled cells revealed that the largest proportion (48%) of GHS-R-expressing cells was colocalized in hypothalamic ARC neurons containing NPY; the percentage of GHS-R-hybridizing cells that expressed GHRH was much lower (Table 1). However, when expressed as a percentage of peptide colocalization, the proportion of ARC and VMN GHRH mRNA-containing neurons co-expressing GHS-R rose to 26% and 21%, respectively. Only a weak hybridization signal for GHS-R was detected in SRIF mRNA-containing neurons in the ARC, VMN and PeV nuclei; the extent of colocalization was lowest for hypothalamic SRIF neurons (Table 1).

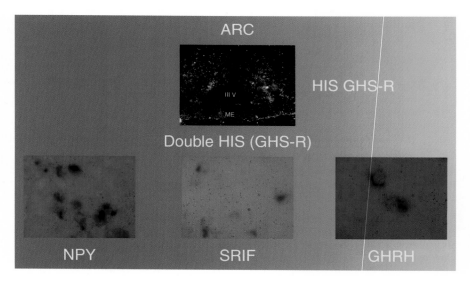

Fig. 5. Photomicrographs of arcuate (ARC) hypothalamic neurons in rat brain sections dually stained for NPY, SRIF or GHRH mRNA (revealed using DIG and stained in brown) and GHS-R mRNA (revealed using autoradiography and detected as silver grain clusters). IIIV, third ventricle; ME, median eminence

Table 1. Estimated percentage of GHRH, SRIF or NPY neurons coexpressing GHS-R mRNA

	Arcuate nucleus	Ventromedial nucleus	Periventricular nucleus
GHRH coexpressing GHS-R	26.9 ± 2.4	21.8 ± 5.1	nd
SRIF coexpressing GHS-R	6.2 ± 2.1	4.3 ± 2.3	5.2 ± 0.2
NPY coexpressing GHS-R	15.9 ± 2.8	nd	nd
GHS-R coexpressing GHRH	7.3 ± 0.9	3.4 ± 2.9	nd
GHS-R coexpressing SRIF	2.6 ± 0.4	1.6 ± 0.8	15.7 ± 3.7
GHS-R coexpressing NPY	29.5 ± 2.1	nd	nd

Values are the mean ± SE of three to four animals per group.
nd: not detected

Discussion

The physiological results reported here clearly demonstrate that ghrelin, administered systemically, causes potent stimulation of spontaneous GH secretion, confirming earlier findings in conscious adult male rats (Seoane et al. 2000; Tolle et al. 2001). In the present study, GH responsiveness to ghrelin was found to be time-dependent, with high GH release observed within five min after injection when ghrelin was administered during a time of a spontaneous GH secretory episode but a markedly attenuated GH response to ghrelin, at five min, when injected during GH trough periods. We have previously shown that the weak GH response to GHRH during GH trough periods is due to antagonism by the cyclical, increased release of endogenous SRIF in the male rat (Tannenbaum and Ling 1984). Indeed, in the present study, immunoneutralization of endogenous SRIF reversed the blunted five-min GH response to ghrelin at trough times, to levels as high as those observed during GH peak periods. These results provide good evidence that SRIF can antagonize ghrelin's GH-releasing activity. Furthermore, our finding that ghrelin effectively stimulates GH secretion in the absence of SRIF indicates that its GH-releasing activity is not dependent on inhibiting endogenous SRIF tone.

It is important to note, however, that full recovery of the GH response to ghrelin during the trough period was evident by 15 min after injection in all groups. This temporal pattern of GH responsiveness to ghrelin differs from that previously found with GHRH, wherein GHRH-induced GH release remained blunted throughout the GH trough period (Tannenbaum and Ling 1984). The present in vivo results, therefore, support the notion that ghrelin is a functional antagonist of SRIF, and they are in conformity with earlier reports demonstrating that GHSs behave as functional antagonists of SRIF activity at the level of the pituitary gland (Smith et al. 1996). The GH response to ghrelin in humans was also shown to be partially refractory to the inhibitory effect of exogenous SRIF (Broglio et al. 2001).

In striking contrast to the effects of anti-SRIF serum, immunoneutralization of endogenous GHRH virtually obliterated the GH responses to ghrelin irrespective of the time of administration, strongly indicating that the GH response to ghrelin in vivo requires an intact GHRH system. This finding is congruent with previous reports indicating that GHS-induced GH release is attenuated by GHRH anti-serum (Clark and Robinson 1989; Tannenbaum and Bowers 2001; Bowers et al. 1991). Indeed, there is convincing evidence that GHSs/ghrelin stimulate GH release via GHRH-dependent pathways. Both GHSs (Dickson et al. 1993) and ghre-lin (Hewson and Dickson 2000) have been shown to activate a subpopulation of hypothalamic arcuate neurons, and GHS-induced c-fos expression was observed in GHRH mRNA-containing cells in the ARC nucleus (Dickson and Luckman 1997). Moreover, GHS administration to conscious sheep provokes the release of GHRH into hypophyseal portal blood but does not influence SRIF release (Guil-laume et al. 1994). Together, these results implicate GHRH neurons as targets for ghrelin. We interpret all these findings to indicate that ghrelin does not act by al-tering hypothalamic SRIF release but rather stimulates GH release via GHRH-de-pendent pathways.

Our dual chromogenic and autoradiographic in situ hybridization experi-ments provide anatomical evidence to support this notion. Quantitative analysis of double-labeled cells revealed that GHRH mRNA-containing neurons in ARC and VMN of the hypothalamus expressed the GHS-R, implying that ghrelin may directly modulate GHRH release into hypophyseal portal blood and thereby in-fluence GH secretion through interaction with the GHS-R on GHRH-containing neurons. A very weak hybridization signal was detected in SRIF mRNA-contain-ing neurons in PeV, the primary source of hypophysiotrophic SRIF neurons pro-jecting to the median eminence (Kawano and Daikoku 1998), suggesting that SRIF cells are not major direct targets for ghrelin's actions on GH. The largest proportion (30 %) of GHS-R-expressing cells was colocalized in hypothalamic ARC neurons containing NPY, one of the most potent orexigenic peptides (Clark et al. 1984; Stanley et al. 1986). This finding is consistent with an earlier report (Willesen et al. 1999), although the percentage of NPY neurons coexpressing GHS-R mRNA in that study was far greater than that found in the present work. In any case, these anatomical findings provide compelling evidence that ghrelin's orexigenic effect is mediated, at least in part, via stimulation of NPY-expressing arcuate neurons. Indeed, centrally administered ghrelin increases hypothalamic NPY mRNA expression (Nakazato et al. 2001; Kamegai et al. 2001; Shintani et al. 2001), and pretreatment with either antiserum to NPY (Nakazato et al. 2001) or specific NPY receptor antagonists (Nakazato et al. 2001; Shintani et al. 2001) sig-nificantly interfered with ghrelin's appetite-stimulating effect. Both centrally (Nakazato et al. 2001) and systemically (Hewson and Dickson 2000) administered ghrelin were shown to induce c-fos expression in a subpopulation of arcuate neu-rons where NPY cells are located; the latter findings suggest that stomach-derived ghrelin may reach hypothalamic sites by penetrating the blood-brain barrier (perhaps due to its octanoyl moiety adding hydrophobicity to the molecule). Fi-nally, it is also possible that ghrelin's actions on GH may be mediated, in part, by NPY, since hypothalamic NPY pathways have been shown to influence GH secre-tion (Rettori et al. 1990; Kamegai et al. 1996).

In summary, the results of the present study demonstrate that: 1) ghrelin, ad-ministered peripherally, exerts potent, time-dependent GH-releasing activity un-der physiological conditions; 2) ghrelin is a functional antagonist of SRIF, but its

GH-releasing activity is not dependent on inhibiting endogenous SRIF release; 3) SRIF antagonizes the actions of ghrelin acting at the level of the pituitary gland; 4) the GH response to ghrelin requires an intact endogenous GHRH system; and 5) hypothalamic ARC GHRH- and NPY-containing neurons, but not PeV SRIF-expressing cells, are major direct targets for ghrelin. The dual action of ghrelin on GH secretion and food intake, in conjunction with the finding that the stomach rather than the hypothalamus is the major anatomic origin of ghrelin, supports the notion that ghrelin may be a critical hormonal signal of nutritional status to the GH neuroendocrine axis, serving to integrate energy balance and the growth process. The challenge ahead is to determine whether stomach ghrelin versus hypothalamic ghrelin, or both, play a physiologically important role in the genesis of GH pulsatility at the level of either the pituitary or hypothalamus under normal conditions, or whether ghrelin's role in GH regulation only becomes more active and more prominent during states of negative energy balance.

Acknowledgments

We thank Drs. Andrew Howard, Kelly Mayo and Robert Steiner for provision of the rat GHS-R cDNA, rat GHRH cDNA, and rat NPY and rat SRIF cDNAs, respectively; Dr. Kang Chang for the gift of human ghrelin; and the National Institute of Diabetes and Digestive and Kidney Diseases for the gift of GH RIA materials. We are grateful to Wendy Gurd, Geneviève Parent, Rachael Eniojukian and Geneviève Toupin for technical assistance, and to Julie Temko for preparation of the manuscript. This work was supported by Grant MT-15440 (to G.S.T.) from the Canadian Institutes of Health Research. G.S.T. is a Chercheur de Carrière of the Fonds de la Recherche en Santé du Québec.

References

Arvat E, Di Vito L, Broglio F, Papotti M, Muccioli G, Dieguez C, Casanueva FF, Deghenghi R, Camanni F, Ghigo E (2000) Preliminary evidence that Ghrelin, the natural GH secretagogue (GHS)-receptor ligand, strongly stimulates GH secretion in humans. J Endocrinol Invest 23: 493–495

Bennett PA, Thomas GB, Howard AD, Feighner SC, Van der Ploeg LHT, Smith RG, Robinson ICAF (1997) Hypothalamic growth hormone secretagogue-receptor (GHS-R) expression is regulated by growth hormone in the rat. Endocrinology 138: 4552–4557

Bowers CY (1999) Growth hormone-releasing peptides. In: Kostyo JL, Goodman HM (eds) Handbook of physiology, Section 7: The endocrine system, Volume V: Hormonal control of growth. Oxford University Press, New York, pp 267–297

Bowers CY, Momany FA, Reynolds GA, Hong A (1984) On the *in vitro* and *in vivo* activity of a new synthetic hexapeptide that acts on the pituitary to specifically release growth hormone. Endocrinology 114: 1537–1545

Bowers CY, Sartor AO, Reynolds GA, Badger TM (1991) On the actions of the growth hormone-releasing hexapeptide, GHRP. Endocrinology 128: 2027–2035

Broglio F, Di Vito L, Gottero C, Prodam F, Benso A, Papotti M, Muccioli G, Deghenghi R, Ghigo E, Arvat, E (2001) The GH-releasing effect of ghrelin, a natural GH secretagogue, is partially refractory to the inhibitory effect of exogenous somatostatin in humans. Prog 83rd Ann Meet Endocrinol Soc OR9-2

Carrel AL, Allen DB (2000) Effects of growth hormone on body composition and bone metabolism. Endocrine 12: 163–172

Clark JT, Kalra PS, Crowley WR, Kalra SP (1984) Neuropeptide Y and human pancreatic polypeptide stimulate feeding behavior in rats. Endocrinology 427–429

Clark RG, Robinson ICAF (1989) Growth hormone responses to multiple injections of a fragment of human growth hormone-releasing factor in conscious male and female rats. J Endocrinol 106: 281–289

Dickson SL, Leng G, Robinson ICAF (1993) Systemic administration of growth hormone-releasing peptide activates hypothalamic arcuate neurons. Neuroscience 53: 303–306

Dickson SL, Luckman SM (1997) Induction of c-*fos* messenger ribonucleic acid in neuropeptide Y and growth hormone (GH)-releasing factor neurons in the rat arcuate nucleus following systemic injection of the GH secretagogue, GH-releasing peptide-6. Endocrinology 138: 771–777

Guan X-M, Yu H, Palyha OC, McKee KK, Feighner SD, Sirinathsinghji DJS, Smith RG, Van der Ploeg LHT, Howard AD (1997) Distribution of mRNA encoding the growth hormone secretagogue receptor in brain and peripheral tissues. Mol Brain Res 48: 23–29

Guillaume V, Magnan E, Cataldi M, Dutour A, Sauze N, Renard M, Razafindraibe H, Conte-Devolx B, Deghenghi R, Lenaerts V, Oliver C (1994) Growth hormone (GH)-releasing hormone secretion is stimulated by a new GH-releasing hexapeptide in sheep. Endocrinology 135: 1073–1076

Hewson AK, Dickson SL (2000) Systemic administration of ghrelin induces Fos and Egr-1 proteins in the hypothalamic arcuate nucleus of fasted and fed rats. J Neuroendocrinol 12: 1047–1049

Howard AD, Feighner SD, Cully DF, Arena JP, Liberator PA, Rosenblum CI, Hamelin M, Hreniuk DL, Palyha OC, Anderson J, Paress PS, Diaz C, Chou M, Liu KK, McKee KK, Pong SS, Chaung LY, Elbrecht A, Dashkevicz M, Heavens R, Rigby M, Sirinathsinghji DJS, Dean DC, Melillo DG, Patchett AA, Nargund R, Griffin PR, Gupta SK, Schaeffer JM, Smith RG, Van der Ploeg LH. (1996) A receptor in pituitary and hypothalamus that functions in growth hormone release. Science 273: 974–977.

Kamegai J, Minami S, Sugihara H, Higuchi H, Wakabayashi I (1996) Growth hormone receptor gene is expressed in neuropeptide Y neurons in hypothalamic arcuate nucleus of rats. Endocrinology 137: 2109–2112

Kamegai J, Tamura H, Shimizu T, Ishii S, Sugihara H, Wakabayashi I (2001) Chronic central infusion of ghrelin increases hypothalamic neuropeptide Y and agouti-related protein mRNA levels and body weight in rats. Diabetes 50: 2438–2443

Kamegai J, Wakabayashi I, Miyamoto K, Unterman TG, Kineman RD, Frohman LA (1998) Growth hormone (GH)-dependent regulation of pituitary GH secretagogue receptor (GHS-R) mRNA levels in the spontaneous dwarf rat. Neuroendocrinology 68: 312–318

Kawano H, Daikoku S (1998) Somatostatin-containing neuron systems in the rat hypothalamus: retrograde tracing and immunohistochemical studies. J Comp Neurol 271: 293–299.

Kojima M, Hosoda H, Date Y, Nakazato M, Matsuo H, Kangawa K (1999) Ghrelin is a growth-hormone-releasing acylated peptide from stomach. Nature 402: 656–660

Korbonits M, Bustin SA, Kojima M, Jordan S, Adams EF, Lowe DG, Kangawa K, Grossman AB (2001) The expression of the growth hormone secretagogue receptor ligand ghrelin in normal and abnormal human pituitary and other neuroendocrine tumors. J Clin Endocrinol Metab 86: 881–887

Lu S, Guan J-L, Wang Q-P, Uehara K, Yamada S, Goto N, Date Y, Nakazato M, Kojima M, Kangawa K, Shioda S (2002) Immunocytochemical observation of ghrelin-containing neurons in the rat arcuate nucleus. Neurosci Lett 321: 157–160

McKee KK, Palyha OC, Feighner SD, Hreniuk DL, Tan CP, Phillips MS, Smith RG, Vanderploeg LHT, Howard AD (1997) Molecular analysis of rat pituitary and hypothalamic growth hormone secretagogue receptors. Mol Endocrinol 11: 415–423

Nakazato M, Murakami N, Date Y, Kojima M, Matsuo H, Kangawa K, Matsukura S (2001) A role for ghrelin in the central regulation of feeding. Nature 409: 194–198

Painson J-C, Tannenbaum GS (1991) Sexual dimorphism of somatostatin and growth hormone-releasing factor signaling in the control of pulsatile growth hormone secretion in the rat. Endocrinology 128: 2858–2866

Rettori V, Milenkovic L, Aguila MC, McCann SM (1990) Physiologically significant effect of neuropeptide Y to suppress growth hormone release by stimulating somatostatin discharge. Endocrinology 126: 2296–2301

Seoane LM, Tovar S, Baldelli R, Arvat E, Ghigo E, Casanueva FF, Dieguez C (2000) Ghrelin elicits a marked stimulatory effect on GH secretion in freely-moving rats. Eur J Endocrinol 143: R7–R9

Shintani M, Ogawa Y, Ebihara K, Aizawa-Abe M, Miyanaga F, Takaya K, Hayashi T, Inoue G, Hosoda K, Kojima M, Kangawa K, Nakao K (2001) Ghrelin, an endogenous growth hormone secretagogue, is a novel orexigenic peptide that antagonizes leptin action through the activation of hypothalamic neuropeptide Y/Y1 receptor pathway. Diabetes 50: 227–232

Smith RG, Cheng K, Pong S-S, Leonard RJ, Cohen CJ, Arena JP, Hickey GJ, Chang CH, Jacks TM, Drisko JE, Robinson ICAF, Dickson SL, Leng G (1996) Mechanism of action of GHRP-6 and nonpeptidyl growth hormone Secretagogue. In: Bercu BB, Walker RF (eds) Growth hormone secretagogues. Springer-Verlag, New York, pp 147–163

Smith RG, Van der Ploeg LHT, Howard AD, Feighner SD, Cheng K, Hickey GJ, Wyvratt Jr. MJ, Fisher MH, Nargund RP, Patchett AA (1997) Peptidomimetic regulation of growth hormone secretion. Endocrinol Rev 18: 621–645

Stanley BG, Kyrkouli SE, Lampert S, Leibowitz SF (1986) Neuropeptide Y chronically injected into the hypothalamus: a powerful neurochemical inducer of hyperphagia and obesity. Peptides 7: 1189–1192.

Takaya K, Ariyasu H, Kanamoto N, Iwakura H, Yoshimoto A, Harada M, Mori K, Komatsu Y, Usui T, Shimatsu A, Ogawa Y, Hosoda K, Akamizu T, Kojima M, Kangawa K, Nakao K (2000) Ghrelin strongly stimulates growth hormone (GH) release in humans. J Clin Endocrinol Metab 85: 4908–4911

Tannenbaum GS, Bowers CY (2001) Interactions of growth hormone secretagogues and growth hormone-releasing hormone/somatostatin. Endocrine 14: 21–27

Tannenbaum GS, Epelbaum J (1999) Somatostatin. In: Kostyo JL, Goodman HM (eds) Handbook of physiology, Section 7: The endocrine system, Volume V: Hormonal control of growth. Oxford University Press, New York, Oxford, pp 221–265

Tannenbaum GS, Lapointe M, Beaudet A, Howard AD (1998) Expression of growth hormone secretagogue-receptors by growth hormone-releasing hormone neurons in the mediobasal hypothalamus. Endocrinology 139: 4420–4423

Tannenbaum GS, Ling N (1984) The interrelationship of growth hormone (GH)-releasing factor and somatostatin in generation of the ultradian rhythm of GH secretion. Endocrinology 115: 1952–1957

Tannenbaum GS, Martin JB (1976) Evidence for an endogenous ultradian rhythm governing growth hormone secretion in the rat. Endocrinology 98: 562–570

Tannenbaum GS, Zhang W-H, Lapointe M, Zeitler P, Beaudet A (1998) Growth hormone-releasing hormone neurons in the arcuate nucleus express both sst1 and sst2 somatostatin receptor genes. Endocrinology 139: 1450–1453

Tolle V, Zizzari P, Tomasetto C, Rio M-C, Epelbaum J, Bluet-Pajot M-T (2001) In vivo and in vitro effects of ghrelin/motilin-related peptide on growth hormone secretion in the rat. Neuroendocrinology 73: 54–61

Tschöp M, Smiley DL, Heiman ML (2000) Ghrelin induces adiposity in rodents. Nature 407: 908–913

Wagner C, Caplan SR, Tannenbaum GS (1998) Genesis of the ultradian rhythm of growth hormone secretion: a new model unifying experimental observations in rats. Am J Physiol 275 (Endocrinol Metab 38) E1046–E1054

Willesen MG, Kristensen P, Romer J (1999) Co-localization of growth hormone secretagogue receptor and NPY mRNA in the arcuate nucleus of the rat. Neuroendocrinology 70: 306–316

Wren AM, Small CJ, Ward HL, Murphy KG, Dakin CL, Taheri S, Kennedy AR, Roberts GH, Morgan DGA, Ghatei MA, Bloom SR (2000) The novel hypothalamic peptide ghrelin stimulates food intake and growth hormone secretion. Endocrinology 141: 4325–4328

Adipose Tissues as Part of the Immune System: Role of Leptin and Cytokines

L. Pénicaud[1], B. Cousin[1], P. Laharrague[1], C. Leloup[1], A. Lorsignol[1], and L. Casteilla[1]

Summary

In addition to its classical role in energy metabolism, there is more and more evidence that adipose tissues could be a player in other physiological processes, including immunity and inflammation. Numerous data have accumulated showing a strong interplay between factors of inflammation (cytokines, adipsin for example) and adipose cells. First, preadipocytes or adipocytes of both peripheral or bone marrow origins are able to synthesise and secrete a variety of inflammatory cytokines. Conversely, some of these factors control adipose cell development and functions. Second, recent papers support the notion that leptin, the main secretory product of adipocytes, is directly involved in the regulation of immune parameters. Even more intriguing is the putative role of leptin in the regulation of hematopoiesis. Third, we have demonstrated that preadipocytes share numerous characteristics with macrophages. Using some of these properties, adipose tissue controls, both directly and indirectly via the brain and the autonomic nervous system, its own development and whole body energy homeostasis.

Introduction

In addition to its classical role in energy metabolism, there is more and more evidence that adipose tissues could be a player in other physiological processes, including immunity and inflammation. Indeed infectious diseases, and more generally inflammation occurring in numerous pathological states such as cancer or AIDS, are associated with cachectic states and decreases in both food intake and body fat. Classic clinical data, as well as more recent experimental ones, suggest that obesity or increased body weight is often concomitant with changes in inflammation or immunity-related parameters (Plotkin et al. 1996: Stallone 1994: Tanaka et al. 1993, 1998). It is well known in clinical practice that obese individuals are more prone to infectious diseases as compared to lean individuals (Marks 1960: Tracey et al. 1971). Both enhanced and decreased body weights are linked to alterations in cytokine levels. Recently, numerous data have accumulated showing a strong interplay between cytokines and adipose cells. These and other observa-

[1]UMR 5018 CNRS-UPS, IFR 31, CHU Rangueil, 1 avenue Jean Poulhès, 31054 Toulouse Cedex, France

Kordon et al.
Brain Somatic Cross-Talk and the
Central Control of Metabolism
© Springer-Verlag Berlin Heidelberg 2002

tions that will be reviewed in the present paper lead to the notion that adipose tissue could be part of the inflammatory and immune systems.

Adipose tissues and the lymphatic system

First, one can point to the strong anatomical link between adipose tissue and lymphoid ganglia in rodents and human beings. Most adipose depots contain at least one lymph node, and nearly all major lymph nodes are embedded in adipose tissue (Kampmeier 1969; Suzuki 1952). Such strong anatomical relationships suggest an interplay between the two structures. In this respect, it has then been demonstrated that signals coming from activated lymph nodes stimulate lipolysis in adipocytes and increase their sensitivity to catecholamines (Pond and Mattacks 1995). The products of lipolysis, mainly fatty acids, may constitute for the activated lymphoid cells a source of energy, but also of constitutive lipids for the synthesis of leukotriens, prostaglandins, and prostacyclins (Ardawi and Newsholme 1985). Furthermore it has been demonstrated that fatty acids can alter lymphocyte proliferation (Buttke 1984; Calder et al. 1992, 1994). Altogether these data are in agreement with the occurrence of changes in lipid metabolism during systemic immune responses.

Adipose tissue as a source of inflammatory factors

Over the last 10 years the notion has emerged that adipose tissue is not only involved in the storage and release of energy but could also be involved in other physiological functions, due to its capabilities in synthesis and secretion. Among the secreted compounds are proteins involved in inflammatory or immune functions (Mohamed-Ali et al. 1998; Ahima and Flier 2000, Fig. 1). Adipsin was one of the first of these factors shown to be synthesised and secreted by adipose tissue (Cook et al. 1985). This molecule is the murine equivalent of the complement factor D, the initial and rate-limiting enzyme of the alternative pathway of complement activation (Taylor et al. 1998). It is also required for the synthesis of acylation-stimulating protein, a protein involved in fat metabolism (Cianflone et al. 1999). Subsequently, other complement proteins have been shown to be expressed by adipose tissue, including AdipoQ, which is structurally similar to its complement, factor C1q (Scherer et al. 1995).

Adipose tissue also produces factors such as leukemia inhibitory factor (LIF), macrophage inhibitory factor (MIF), macrophage colony-stimulating factor (MCSF), and transforming growth factor β (Coppack 2001). Furthermore preadipocytes and adipocytes of both peripheral or bone marrow origins are able to synthesise and secrete a variety of inflammatory cytokines, including TNFα, interleukin –1 and –6 (Mohamed-Ali et al. 1998; Laharrague et al. 2000). All these pro-inflammatory cytokines are well known for their involvement in the host defence. More recently, it has been demonstrated that adipocytes have the capacity to secrete chemokines (IL-8, macrophage inflammatory protein-1α and monocyte chemotactic protein-1), a group of low molecular weight peptides that

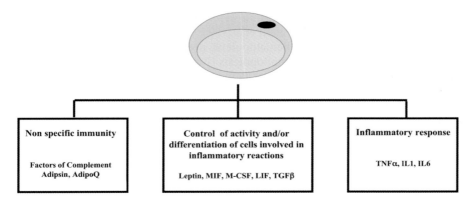

Fig. 1. Adipocyte as a secretory cell. Adipose tissue is able to synthesise and secrete numerous factors and cytokines involved in inflammatory reactions and immune responses.

play the role of inflammatory mediators, mainly by regulating leukocyte migration (Zlotnik et al. 1999; Gerhardt et al. 2001). It has to be emphasized that, even if the synthesis and production of these factors by a cell are not very important, due to the mass of adipose tissues in the whole body, adipose tissue could be one of the main sources of cytokines. This fact has been demonstrated for adipsin.

Leptin and the inflammatory response

The main protein secreted by adipose tissue is leptin, the product of the *ob* gene. Leptin is a peptide hormone mainly involved in the regulation of body fat mass by acting in the central nervous system to regulate both food intake and energy expenditure (Friedman and Halaas 1998; Zhang et al. 1994). The leptin receptor is a cytokine, like receptors sharing signaling capacities of IL-6 receptors (Baumann et al. 1996). This homology leads to works aimed at identifying the relationships between leptin and inflammatory parameters. One of the first links was the demonstration that endotoxin administration induces anorexia, together with an increased plasma leptin level (Grunfeld et al. 1996; Sarraf et al. 1997; Faggioni et al. 1998; Finck et al. 1998). Recent papers support the notion that leptin itself is directly involved in the regulation of immune parameters and hematopoiesis (Fantuzzi and Faggioni 2000). The long form leptin receptor is expressed on different lympho-hematopoietic cells (Bennett et al. 1996; Cioffi et al. 1996; Lord et al. 1998). Leptin enhances the production of oxidative species by neutrophils and induces the secretion of IL-1 receptor antagonist in monocytes (Caldefie-Chezet et al. 2001; Gabay et al. 2001). Furthermore, it acts directly on T cell response by increasing their activation and proliferation. Leptin increases secretion of Th1 cytokines whereas it inhibits those of Th2, both in mice and humans (Lord et al. 1998; Martin-Romero et al. 2000). It also stimulates proliferation of monocytes and induces their production of IL-6 and TNFα (Santos-Alvarez et al. 1999). In *db/db* obese mice, in which the leptin receptor is mutated, lymphocyte number is reduced (Bennett et al. 1996). In addition in *ob/ob* mice with an abnormal leptin, cell-mediated immunity is altered (Chandra 1980).

As previously underlined, the leptin receptor is present on hematopoietic stem cells and hepatic foetal cells (Bennett et al. 1996; Cioffi et al. 1996). In rodents, leptin increases proliferation of hematopoietic progenitors and enhances granulopoiesis, erythropoiesis and lymphopoiesis (Bennett et al. 1996). Along this line, we have been among the first to demonstrate that human bone marrow adipocytes synthesise high levels of leptin (Laharrague et al. 1998). We have shown that marrow adipocytes are in close contact to hematopoietic stem cells and that leptin is able to engage these cells towards the monocytes/macrophages cell lineage (Laharrague et al. 2000).

Macrophage-like activity of adipose cells

We have recently demonstrated that preadipocytes share numerous characteristics with macrophages. Thus, proliferating preadipocytes (cell lines and primary cultures), like macrophages, are able to phagocyte and kill microorganisms (Cousin et al. 1999). In addition preadipocytes as well as adipocytes express MOMA-2, a marker of monocyte/macrophage lineage, although they are negative for specific mature macrophage marker (F4/80). These features vary with pathological situations such as inflammation and obesity and depend on the fat pads' localisation (Cousin et al. 2001; Villena et al. 2001). Thus, both phagocytic and candidacical activities are enhanced by thioglycollate treatment in control mice. In *ob/ob* mice, there is a severe defect in anti-microbial activity of both macrophages and preadipocytes. Others have also demonstrated an alteration in macrophage functions, such as microbicidal activity, cytokine secretion, and radical oxygen species production in genetically obese mice (Lee et al. 1999; Loffreda et al. 1998). Furthermore, mice deficient in Mac-1, another marker of monocytes/macrophages, develop an unexpected obesity (Dong et al. 1997).

These results suggest that preadipocytes could function as macrophages and raise the possibility of direct involvement of adipose tissue in inflammatory processes.

Role of cytokines in energy metabolism

Via the secretion of the different cytokines and chemokines cited above, adipose tissue controls its own development and, more generally, energy metabolism, either by direct action (paracrine and autocrine effects) or indirectly by acting on the brain (endocrine effects; Fig. 2).

Direct effect on adipose tissue

Most of the cytokines produced by adipose tissue have metabolic action on adipose tissue itself (Coppack 2001). Thus TNFα and IL-6 inhibit lipoprotein lipase; the former also stimulates hormone-sensitive lipase. TNFα also downregulates insulin- stimulated glucose uptake. All these effects tend to decrease fat mass.

Furthermore, TNFα induces apoptosis and de-differentiation of adipocytes in vitro (Fig. 3; Pénicaud et al. 2000). Chemokines such as IL-8 inhibit adipocyte differentiation and enhance leptin secretion (Gerhardt et al. 2001).

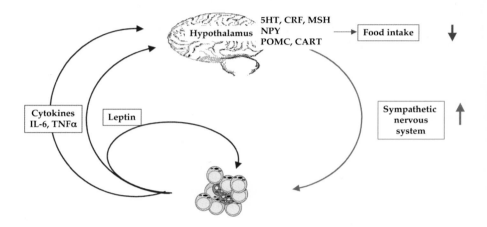

Fig. 2. Feedback loop between adipose tissue and the brain. The cytokines produced by adipose tissue (leptin, TNFα, IL-6) can act on adipose tissue either directly (autocrine and paracrine effects) or indirectly (endocrine effect) via the brain. Through their action on the central nervous system, they are involved in the regulation of food intake and on the activity of the autonomic nervous system, thus on whole body energy metabolism.

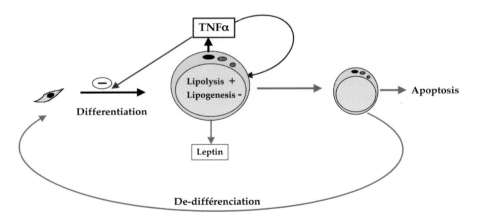

Fig. 3. The role of TNFα on adipose cell development. TNFα can act both on adipocyte metabolism (lipolysis and lipogenesis), thus inducing cell dedifferentiation, and on adipocyte development (induction of apoptosis, inhibition of cell differentiation).

Indirect effect via the brain

The effects of leptin on the brain, and thus on food intake and energy expenditure, have been extensively reviewed (Campfield et al. 1996; Friedman and Halaas 1998). Apart from leptin, it is well known that numerous cytokines, including those produced by adipose tissue (IL-6 and TNFα), inhibit feeding and increase sympathetic nervous system activity (Konsman and Dantzer 2001; Langhans 2000; Plata-Salaman 1996). This fact is the basis of the anorexia occurring during infection. Indeed, most cytokines can reach the central nervous system receptors through circumventricular organs and through active or passive transports. These cytokines, like leptin, directly alter hypothalamic neuronal activity implicated in the control of food intake. Numerous data demonstrate changes in neuromediators and neuropeptide contents in the different nuclei involved in both food intake and autonomic nervous system regulation (Konsman and Dantzer 2001; Langhans 2000).

By altering the autonomic nervous system, leptin and other cytokines will change whole body energy metabolism and adipose tissue metabolism and development (Pénicaud et al. 1996, 2000). Thus, its is well known that one of the main regulators of lipolysis is norepinephrine. Furthermore, we have shown that the sympathetic nervous system negatively controls proliferation of preadipocytes, i.e., an increased sympathetic tone induced by cytokines will tend to inhibit white adipocyte proliferation and thus adipose tissue development (Cousin et al. 1993).

Via these direct or indirect effects, cytokines could contribute to the important plasticity of adipose tissue by modulating cell size and number and, as a consequence, could decrease the fat mass of the individual (Casteilla et al. 1996).

Conclusion

Altogether, these data demonstrate a very close relationship between adipose tissues and inflammation, immunity and hematopoiesis. This finding opens a new field of investigation for the comprehension of the interplay between these physiological processes as well as that of the relationship between metabolic and inflammatory/immunological diseases.

Acknowledgements

This work has been sustained over the year by the CNRS, the University Paul Sabatier Toulouse and the French Ministry for Research.

References

Ahima RS, Flier JS (2000) Adipose tissue as an endocrine organ. Trends Endocrinol Metab. 11: 327–332

Ardawi MSM, Newsholme EA (1985) Metabolism in lymphocytes and its importance in the immune response. Essays Biochem 21: 1–43

Baumann H, Morella KK, White DW, Dembski M, Bailon PS, Kim H, Lai CF, Tartaglia LA (1996) The full-length leptin receptor has signaling capabilities of interleukin 6-type cytokine receptors. Proc Natl Acad Sci USA 93: 8374–8378

Bennett BD, Solar GP, Yuan JQ, Mathias J, Thomas GR, Matthews W (1996) A role for leptin and its cognate receptor in hematopoiesis. Curr Biol 6: 1170–1180

Buttke TM (1984) Inhibition of lymphocyte proliferation by free fatty acids. 1. Differential effects on mouse B and T lymphocytes. Immunology. 53: 235–242

Caldefie-Chezet F, Poulin A, Tridon A, Sion B, Vasson MP (2001) Leptin: a potential regulator of polymorphonuclear neutrophil bactericidal action? J Leukoc Biol 69: 414–418

Calder PC, Bevan SJ, Newsholme EA (1992) The inhibition of T-lymphocyte proliferation by fatty acids is via an eicosanoid-independent mechanism. Immunology 75: 108–115

Calder PC, Yaqoob P, Harvey DJ, Watts A, Newsholme EA (1994) Incorporation of fatty acids by concanavalin A-stimulated lymphocytes and the effect on fatty acid composition and membrane fluidity. Biochem J 300: 509–518

Campfield LA, Smith FJ, Burn P (1996) The OB protein (leptin) pathway. A link between adipose tissue mass and central neural networks. Horm Metab Res 28: 619–632

Casteilla L, Cousin B, Viguerie-Bascands N, Larrouy D, Pénicaud L (1996) Hétérogénéité et plasticité des tissus adipeux. Médecine et Sciences 10: 1099–1106

Chandra RK (1980) Cell-mediated immunity in genetically obese (C57BL/6J ob/ob) mice. Am J Clin Nutr 33: 13–16

Cianflone K, Maslowska M, Sniderman AD (1999) Acylation stimulating protein (ASP), an adipocyte autocrine: new directions. Semin Cell Dev Biol 10: 31 –41

Cioffi J, Shafer A, Zupancic T, Smithbur J, Mikhail A, Platika D, Snodgrass H (1996) Novel B219/OB receptor isoforms: possible role of leptin in hematopoiesis and reproduction. Nature Med 2: 585–589

Cook KS, Groves DL, Min HY, Spiegelman BM (1985) A developmentally regulated mRNA from 3T3 adipocytes encodes a novel serine protease homologue. Proc Natl Acad Sci 82: 64980–6484

Coppack SW (2001) Pro-inflammatory cytokines and adipose tissue. Proc Nutr Soc 60: 349–356

Cousin B, Casteilla L, Lafontan M, Ambid L, Langin D, Berthault MF, Pénicaud L (1993). Local sympathetic denervation of white adipose tissue in rats induces preadipocyte proliferation whithout noticeable change in metabolism. Endocrinology 133: 2255–2262

Cousin B, Munoz O, André M, Fontanilles AM, Dani C, Cousin J.L, Laharrague P, Casteilla L, Pénicaud L (1999). A role for preadipocytes as macrophage-like cells. FASEB J 13: 305–312

Cousin B, André M, Casteilla L, Pénicaud L (2001). Altered macrophage-like functions of preadipocytes in inflammation and genetic obesity. J Cell Physiol 186: 380–386

Dong ZM, Gutierrez-Ramos JC, Coxon A, Mayadas TN, Wagner DD (1997) A new class of obesity genes encodes leukocytes adhesion receptors. Proc Natl Acad Sci USA 94: 7526–7530

Faggioni R, Fantuzzi G, Fuller J, Dinarello CA, Feingold KR, Grunfeld C (1998) IL-1 beta mediates leptin induction during inflammation. Am J Physiol. 43 : R204–R208

Fantuzzi G, Faggioni R (2000) Leptin in the regulation of immunity, inflammation, and hematopoiesis. J Leukoc Biol 68 : 437–446

Finck BN, Kelley KW, Dantzer R, Johnson RW (1998) In vivo and in vitro evidence for the involvement of tumor necrosis factor-alpha in the induction of leptin by lipopolysaccharide. Endocrinol. 139: 2278–2283

Friedman JM, Halaas JL (1998) Leptin and the regulation of body weight in mammals. Nature 395 : 763–770

Gabay C, Dreyer M, Pelligrinelli N, Chicheportiche R, Meier CA (2001) Leptin directly induces the secretion of interleukin 1 receptor antagonist in human monocytes. J Clin Endocrinol Metab 86: 783–791

Gerhardt CC, Romero IA, Cancello R, Camoin L, Strosberg AD (2001) Chemokines control fat accumulation and leptin secretion by cultured human adipocytes. Molec Cell Endocrinol 175: 81–92

Grunfeld C, Zhao C, Fuller J, Pollock A, Moser A, Friedman J, Feingold KR (1996) Endotoxin and cytokines induce expression of leptin, the *ob* gene product, in hamsters. A role for leptin in the anorexia of infection. J Clin Invest 97: 2152–2157

Kampmeier OF (1969) Evolution and comparative morphology of the lymphatic system. Thomas, C.C., Springfield, IL, pp. 412–517

Konsman JP, Dantzer R (2001) How the immune and nervous system interact during disease-associated anorexia. Nutrition 17: 664–668

Laharrague P, Larrouy D, Fontanilles AM, Truel N, Campfield A, Tenenbaum R, Galitzky J, Corberand JX, Penicaud L, Casteilla L (1998) High expression of leptin by human bone marrow adipocytes in primary culture. FASEB J. 12 : 747–752

Laharrague P, Oppert JM, Brousset P, Charlet JP, Campfield A, Fontanilles AM, Guy-Grand B, Corberand JX, Penicaud L, Casteilla L (2000) High concentration of leptin stimulates myeloid differentiation from human bone marrow CD34+ progenitors: potential involvement in leukocytosis of obese subjects. Int J Obes 24: 1212–1216

Langhans W (2000) Anorexia of infection: current prospects. Nutrition 16: 996–1005

Lee FYJ, Li Y, Yang EK, Yang SQ, Lin HZ, Trush MA, Dannenberg AJ, Diehlv AM (1999) Phenotypic abnormalities in macrophages from leptin-deficient, obese mice. Am J Physiol. 276: C386–C394

Loffreda S, Yang SQ, Lin HZ, Karp CL, Brengman ML, Wang DJ, Klein AS, Bulkley GB, Bao C, Noble PW, Lane MD, Diehl AM (1998) Leptin regulates proinflammatory immune responses. FASEB J 12: 57–65

Lord GM, Matarese G, Howard JK, Baker RJ, Bloom SR, Lechler RI (1998) Leptin modulates the T-cell immune response and reverses starvation-induced immunosuppression. Nature. 394: 897–901

Marks HH (1960) Influence of obesity on morbidity and mortality. Bull NY Acad Med 36: 296–312

Martin-Romero C, Santos-Alvarez J, Goberna R, Sanchez-Margalet V (2000) Human leptin enhances activation and proliferation of human circulating T lymphocytes. Cell Immunol 199: 15–24

Mohamed-Ali V, Pinckney JH, Coppack SW (1998) Adipose tissue as an endocrine and paracrine organ. Int J Obes. 22: 1145–1158

Pénicaud L, Cousin B, Leloup C, AtefN, Casteilla L, Ktorza A (1996) Changes in autonomic nervous system and consecutive hyperinsulinemia: respective roles in the development of obesity in rodents. Diabetes Metabolism 22: 15–24

Pénicaud L, Cousin B, Leloup C, Lorsignol A, Casteilla L (2000) The autonomic nervous system, adipose tissue plasticity and energy balance. Nutrition 16: 903–908

Plata-Salaman CR (1996) Anorexia during acute and chronic disease. Nutrition 12: 69

Plotkin BJ, Paulson D, Chelich A, Jurak D, Cole J, Kasimo J, Burdick JR, Casteeel (1996) Immune responsiveness in a rat model for type II diabetes (Zucker rat, fa/fa): susceptibility to Candida albicans infection and leucocyte function.J Med Microbiol 44: 277–283

Pond CM, Mattacks CA (1995) Interactions between adipose tissue around lymph nodes and lymphoid cells in vitro. J Lipid Res 36: 2219–2231

Santos-Alvarez J, Goberna R, Sanchez-Margalet V (1999) Human leptin stimulates proliferation and activation of human circulating monocytes. Cell Immunol 194: 6–11

Sarraf P, Frederich RC, Turner EM, Ma G, Jaskowiak NT, Rivet DJ, Flier JS, Lowell BB, Fraker DL, Alexander HR (1997) Multiple cytokines and acute inflammation raise mouse leptin levels: potential role in inflammatory anorexia. J Exp Med 185: 171–175

Scherer PE, Williams S, Fogliano M, Baldini G, Lodish HF (1995) A novel serum protein similar to C1q, produced exclusively in adipocytes. J Biol Chem 270: 26746–26749

Stallone DD (1994) The influence of obesity and its treatment on the immune system. Nutr Rev 52: 37–50

Suzuki T (1952) Histological studies on lymphatic apparatus in human adipose tissue. Acta Sch Med Univ Kyoto. 30: 174–182

Tanaka S, Inoue S, Isoda F, Waseda M, Ishihara M, Yamakawa T, Sugiyama A, Takamura Y, Okuda K (1993) Impaired immunity in obesity suppressed but reversible lymphocyte responsiveness. Int J Obes 17: 631–636

Tanaka S, Isoda F, Yamakawa T, Ishihara M, Sekihara H (1998) T Lymphopenia in genetically obese rats. Clin Immunol Immunopathol 86: 219–225

Taylor P, Botto M, Walport M (1998) The complement system. Curr Biol 8: R259–R261

Tracey VV, Dew C, Harper JR (1971) Obesity and respiratory infection in infants and young children. Br Med J 1: 17–19

Villena JA, Cousin B, Pénicaud L, Casteilla L (2001) Adipose tissues display differential phagocytic and microbicidal activities depending on their localization. Int J Obes Relat Metab Disord 25: 1275–80

Zhang Y, Proenca R, Maffei M, Barone M, Leopold L, Friedman JM (1994) Positional cloning of the mouse *obese* gene and its human homologue. Nature 372: 425–432

Zlotnik A, Morales J, Hedrick JA (1999) Recent advances in chemokines and chemokines receptors. Crit Rev Immunol 19: 1–47

Regulation of Body Weight Homeostasis During Pregnancy and Lactation

M. C. García[1], R. M. Señaris[1], J. E. Caminos[1], M. Lopez[1], R. Nogueiras[1],
O. Gualillo[1], F. Casanueva[1], and C. Diéguez[1]

Summary

Pregnancy is a hypermetabolic state in which a great increase in maternal body
fat and weight occurs, mostly in the final trimester of gestation, and it is associated with relevant neuroendocrine changes as adaptations to the new hormonal
status. Data gleaned over the last few years have allowed the characterization of
different central and peripheral signals involved in the regulation of body weight
homeostasis.

Serum leptin levels were significantly increased during rat gestation. Leptin
mRNA levels in both the adipose tissue and placenta were higher as pregnancy
progressed, suggesting a role for both tissues in the hyperproduction of leptin.
This paradoxical increase in leptin concentration during gestation suggests that a
physiological state of leptin resistance may exist at the hypothalamic level that
may explain the hyperphagia observed in pregnant rats. A specific reduction of
the mRNA levels encoding the leptin receptor isoform Ob-Rb in the hypothalamus of pregnant rats in comparison to non-pregnant animals suggests that, during pregnancy, the hypothalamus shows a physiological resistance to the high levels of leptin due, at least in part, to a decrease in the expression of the long, biologically active form of the leptin receptor (Ob-Rb). During lactation an increased expression of some of the short forms of the leptin receptor (Ob-Re and
Ob-Rf) was found. This increase could contribute to the hyperphagia present
during lactation. Finally, Neuropeptide (NPY) mRNA levels in the arcuate nucleus
were increased during pregnancy and lactation whereas melanin-concentrating
hormone (MCH) and preprorexin levels were decreased. Therefore, it is possible
that NPY could also be one of the adaptive mechanisms that take place during
pregnancy and lactation in order to meet increased metabolic requirements.

Introduction

Pregnancy is a hypermetabolic state in which a great increase in maternal body
fat and weight occurs, mostly in the final trimester of gestation, and it is associated with relevant neuroendocrine changes as adaptations to the new hormonal

---

[1]Department of Physiology and Medicine, Faculty of Medicine, University of Santiago de Compostela, Spain

Kordon et al.
Brain Somatic Cross-Talk and the
Central Control of Metabolism
© Springer-Verlag Berlin Heidelberg 2002

status. Hypermetabolic changes also occur in the fetus. There is no increase in energetic efficiency in pregnancy, and the energy balance becomes positive primarily due to an increase in food intake, which is necessary to prevent the depletion of maternal energy stores. In humans and some other species, maternal fat accumulates during gestation and is used during lactation (Richard and Trayhurn 1985). Data gleaned over the last few years have allowed the characterization of different central and peripheral signals involved in the regulation of body weight homeostasis (Friedman and Halaas 1998; Casanneva and Dieguez 1999; Flier 1994). In this review we will summarize the role played by leptin and some orexigenic signals in the adaptive mechanisms that take place during pregnancy and lactation in order to meet increased metabolic demands.

Leptin in Pregnancy and Lactation

In humans, there is a general and undisputed pattern of leptin change, i.e, leptin increases at least two-fold at midpregnancy, followed by a decrease just before parturition (Lage et al. 1999). In gestational women, leptin increases in the first trimester of pregnancy, before any major changes in body fat and resting metabolic rate occur. The increase is also unrelated to fetal growth. Immediately before delivery, leptin levels undergo a dramatic drop, returning to the levels in non-pregnant women 24 hours before delivery (Lage et al. 1999). There is no clear explanation for the role of the increased leptin in human pregnancy or the mechanism for these changes. As the human placenta is a source of leptin it has been suggested that maternal leptin levels are derived from this organ (Casanueva and dieguez, 1999). The placenta also expresses the leptin receptors, indicating that the placenta itself may be a target for leptin action (Señarís et al. 1997; Masazaki et al. 1997). In any case, the human placenta is a complex organ with a variety of encoded and expressed neuroendocrine systems; therefore the presence of leptin with specific regulatory systems would not be surprising.

Elevated levels of leptin in serum during pregnancy in rats have been reported by some groups (Kawai et al. 1997; Chien et al. 1997; Gracia et al. 2000; Gavrilova et al. 1997; Tomimatsu et al. 1997; Amico et al. 1998). We found increased expression of leptin mRNA in both the adipose tissue and placenta during gestation (Fig. 1). The discrepancy between these data and those previously reported by other authors (Kawai et al. 1997; Gavrilova et al. 1997) who suggested that leptin is not expressed, in rat placenta, could be due to the different methodology employed, since in other studies leptin mRNA levels were measured by Northern blot whereas we used a more sensitive technique, RT-PCR. Our data do not allow us to determine the relative contribution of adipose tissue and placenta to the hyperleptinemia present in pregnant animals, but the similar pattern of leptin mRNA overexpression in both tissues suggests that both of them could be a source of leptin in this state. Furthermore, the overproduction of Ob-Re by the placenta, which results in large amounts of a circulating form of a leptin-binding protein as reported by others (Gavrilova et al. 1997), would also contribute to maintaining this hyperleptinemia.

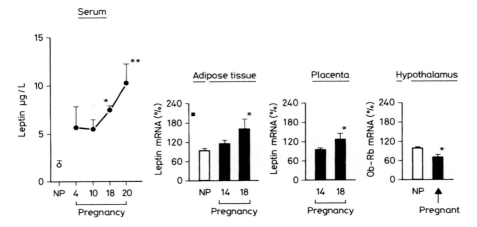

Fig. 1. Serum leptin levels, densitometric analysis of leptin mRNA in adipose tissue and placenta and hypothalamic mRNA levels of Ob-Rb during pregnancy in the rat. Values are expressed as mean ± S.E.M. *p<0.05; **p<0.01. NP, not pregnant.

Although the precise mechanisms by which leptin acts are still unknown, it binds to leptin receptors mainly in the hypothalamus to reduce food intake and increase energy expenditure (Friedman and Halaas 1998; Tartaglia 1997). It is thought that these effects of leptin are mediated by the long isoform of the leptin receptor (Ob-Rb), which contains the full intracellular domain. The function of the other, shorter subtypes is not completely understood. Ob-Ra, which is predominant in all peripheral tissues, is capable of leptin-mediated signalling but much less effectively than the full-length receptor (Murakami et al. 1997). This isoform, together with the other short subtypes, could function as a specific transport system for leptin, as these subtypes are present in high amounts in the choroid plexus and in brain microvessels (Tartaglia 1997; Murakami et al. 1997; Tartaglia et al. 1995; Lee et al. 1996; Cioffi et al. 1996). On the other hand Ob-Re, which is spliced in front of the transmembrane domain, might be a soluble binding protein for leptin (Lee et al. 1996). The other short isoforms could behave as functional antagonists by sequestering leptin and preventing its binding to the Ob-Rb subtype (White et al. 1997). To establish whether the leptin-resistant state of pregnancy could be mediated by changes in the pattern of expression of the long and short forms of the leptin receptor, we determined the levels of expression of the different isoforms in the hypothalamus. We found a significant reduction of the mRNA encoding the fully active form of the leptin receptor (Ob-Rb) in the hypothalamus of pregnant rats in comparison to non-pregnant animals (Fig. 1), whereas no changes were found in the short forms (Gracia et al. 2000). This specific down regulation of the Ob-Rb at the hypothalamic level would explain, at least partially, the state of leptin resistance during pregnancy. However, our data do not allow us to identify whether these changes are specific to some subsets of hypothalamic neurons or are a generalized phenomenon within the hypothalamus.

During lactation, serum leptin concentration returned to the levels found in non-pregnant rats. The energy demand in this state is very high and in met primarily by increased food intake, although there is some mobilization of reserves, especially adipose tissue lipids (Barber et al. 1997). The factors responsible for the massive increase in appetite during lactation remain poorly understood. Serum leptin levels have been shown to be similar in lactating and in non-pregnant animals (Chien et al. 1997; Gracia et al. 2000). Furthermore, we did not observe any change in the hypothalamic expression levels of the long form of the leptin receptor (Ob-Rb) but very interestingly, the levels of the mRNAs of the short forms Ob-Re and Ob-Rf were found to be elevated during lactation (Fig. 2). As previously stated, it is likely that Ob-Re encodes a soluble binding protein. In most peptide hormone/binding protein systems, such as growth hormone, with which leptin exhibits striking similarities, the bound form of the hormone is unable to bind and activate its receptor. In such a case the binding protein would act as an inhibitor of the hormone action. Assuming that the leptin-binding protein would inhibit leptin signalling, the higher levels of Ob-Re mRNA, together with a higher expression of a short, biologically inactive form (Ob-Rf) in the hypothalamus of rats during lactation, would cause leptin resistance that could also contribute to the hyperphagia observed in this state.

In summary, pregnant rats exhibited a marked hyperleptinemia associated with an increase in leptin mRNA levels in both adipose tissue and placenta. Therefore, the hyperphagia observed during pregnancy could be due to a specific decrease of the long, fully active form of the leptin receptor (Ob-Rb) at the hypothalamic level. On the other hand, an increase in the levels of the soluble binding protein of the leptin receptor (Ob-Re), together with an increased expression of one of the short, likely inactive forms of the receptor (Ob-Rf), could be responsible for the increased food intake present during lactation. In conclusion, these data indicate the existence of different regulatory mechanisms on leptin receptor gene expression during pregnancy and lactation that should allow a greater un-

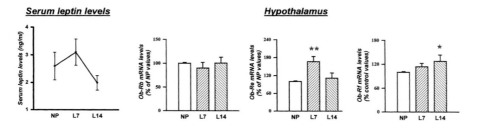

Fig. 2. Serum leptin levels and densitometric analysis of hypothalamic mRNA levels of different isoforms of the leptin receptor during lactation in the rat. Values are expressed as mean ± S.E.M. *p<0.05; **p<0.01.

derstanding of the adaptative responses that take place in these physiological settings.

Orexigenic Signals During Pregnancy and Lactation

Neuropeptide Y (NPY), melanin-concentrating hormone (MCH) and orexins are involved in the control of food intake (Kalra et al. 1999; Qu et al. 1996; Sakurai et al. 1998). These neuropeptides have been reported to display orexigenic functions and to be regulated by leptin levels (Kalra et al. 1999; Qu et al. 1996; Sakurai et al. 1998; Edwards et al. 1999; Lopez et al. 2000). Nutritional status can alter the expression of these appetite-regulating peptides, and therefore they were good candidates as possible mediators of the hyperphagia present during pregnacy and lactation.

NPY has been demonstrated to greatly increase food intake in the arcuate nucleus of the hypothalamus, and the nerve fibers from this nucleus project into various hypothalamic sites that are implicated in the regulation of feeding behaviour (Kalra et al. 1999). We found that NPY mRNA levels were increased in the arcuate nucleus of the hypothalamus in pregnant and in lactating rats. In contrast, no change was observed in the dorsomedia nucleus. Therefore the increase in NPY-gene expression in the arcuate nucleus during pregnancy and lactation may be partly responsible for the hyperphagia seen in these two models of physiological hyperphagia. Surprisingly the hypothalamic levels of the two other orexigenic genes assessed, prepro-orexin and MCH, were markedly reduced during pregnancy and to a lesser extent in lactation. These results indicate that, during gestation, there is a strong inhibitory effect on their expression and that they are not apparently involved in the increased food intake seen in pregnancy and lactation.

Finally, we characterized the expression of the newly discovered hormone, ghrelin (Kojima et al. 1999), in placenta as well as assessing the changes during pregnancy in the rat. The first evidence that the ghrelin system could be involved in the regulation of body weight homeostasis was obtained assessing the effects of different synthetic growth hormone secretagogues (GHSs) on food intake. Thus, it was found that these peptides exerted a significant increase in food intake when administered i.c.v. to experimental animals (Torsello et al. 1998; Okada et al. 1996). Further indirect evidence was obtained with in situ hybridization studies that revealed that the GHS-R gene was expressed in different hypothalamic regions involved in the regulation of energy balance (Willesen et al. 1999). Once the endogenous ligand of the GHS-R, named ghrelin, was discovered, the possible role of this peptide in the regulation of food intake received considerable attention. Data obtained recently by several research groups have shown that exogenous ghrelin administration induces a positive energy balance in rodents by decreasing fat utilization without significantly changing energy expenditure or locomotor activity (Tschop et al. 2000). The effect of ghrelin appears to be exerted at the central level and its chronic administration is associated with metabolic changes that lead to an efficient metabolic state resulting in increased body weight and fat mass (Horvath et al. 2001). Although the mechanisms by which

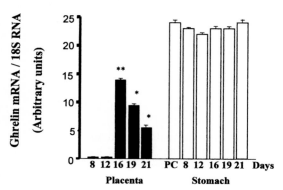

Fig. 3. Densitometric analysis of gastric and placental ghrelin mRNA expression throughout pregnancy. ** p<0.01; * p<0.05.

ghrelin exerts these effects on body weight homeostasis are still unclear, they appear to be unrelated to its stimulatory effect on GH synthesis and secretion (Dieguez and Casanueva 2001).

We found that ghrelin messenger RNA and ghrelin peptide are present in human as well as in rat placentae. In human placenta ghrelin was detected by PCR at both first trimester and at termini. While ghrelin was easily identified by immunohistochemistry at first trimester, it was not detected by immunohistochemistry at termini. Ghrelin was also identified in a cultured human choriocarcinoma cell line, BeWo cells. Ghrelin was found in the cytoplasm of labyrinth trophoblast of rat placenta whereas other placental cell types seem to be negative for ghrelin immunostaining (Gualillo et al. 2001).

Moreover, placental ghrelin mRNA in pregnant rats showed a characteristic profile of expression, being practically undetectable during early pregnancy, with a sharp peak of expression at day 16 and decreasing in the latter stages of gestation (Fig. 3). In contrast, we failed to find any change in stomach-derived ghrelin mRNA levels or in circulating levels (Gualillo et al. 2001). In any case, the finding that ghrelin in placenta shows a period of pregnancy-related expression, a fact not paralleled in gastric tissue, suggests how, more than a tissue reporter, ghrelin may have physiological functions in gestation. Whether alterations in ghrelin-gene expression could be involved in intrauterine growth retardation needs to be established. Interestingly, the ghrelin receptor is located close to the map position of the Brachmann-de-Lange syndrome, a pre- and postnatal growth deficiency (Aqua et al. 1995).

Acknowledgements

This study was supported by grants from the CICYT and the Xunta de Galicia. OG is a recipient of a Spanish Ministry of Health (Institute of Health Carlos III and Fondo de Investigación Sanitaria) contract of research. JEC is a recipient of a predoctoral grant from University of Santiago de Compostela.

References

Amico JA, Thomas A, Crowley RS, Burmeister LA (1998) Concentrations of leptin in the serum of pregnant, lactating, and cycling rats and of leptin messenger ribonucleic acid in rat placental tissue. Life Sci 63:1387–1395.

Aqua MS, Rizzu P, Lindsay EA, Shafer LG, Zackai EH, Overhauser J, Baldini A (1995) Duplication of 3q syndrome: molecular delineation of the critical region. Am J Med Genet 55:33–37.

Barber MC, Clegg RA, Travers MT, Vernon RG (1997) Lipid metabolism in the lactating mammary gland. Biochim Biophys Acta 1347:101–126.

Casanueva FF, Dieguez C (1999) Neuroendocrine regulation and actions of leptin. Front Neuroendocrinol 20:317–363.

Chien EK, Hara M, Rovard M, Yano H, Phillipe M, Polonsky KS, Bell GI (1997) Increase in serum leptin and uterine leptin receptor messenger RNA levels during pregnancy in rats. Biochem Biophys Res Commun 237:476–480.

Cioffi JA, Shafer AW, Zupancic TJ, Smith-Gbur J, Mikhail A, Platika D, Snodgrass HR (1996). Novel B219/OB receptor isoforms: possible role of leptin in hematopoiesis and reproduction. Nature Med 2:585–589.

Dieguez C, Casanueva FF (2001) Ghrelin: a step forward in the understanding of somatotroph cell function and growth regulation. Eur J Endocrinol 142:413–417.

Edwards CM, Abusnana S, Sunter D, Murphy KG, Ghatei MA, Bloom SR (1999) The effects of orexins on food intake: comparisons with neuropeptide Y, melanin-concentarting hormone and galanin. J. Endocrinol 160:R7-R12.

Flier JS (1994) Leptin expression and action: new experimental paradigms. Proc Natl Acad Sci USA 94:4242–4245.

Friedman JM, Halaas JL (1998) Leptin and the regulation of body weight in mammals. Nature 395:763–770.

Gavrilova O, Barr V, Marcus-Samuels B, Reitman M (1997) Hyperleptinemia of pregnancy associated with the appearance of a circulating form of the leptin receptor. J Biol Chem 272:30546–30551.

Gracia MC, Casanueva FF, Dieguez C, Señaris RM (2000) Gestational profile of leptin messenger ribonucleuc acid (mRNA) content in the placenta and adipose tissue in the rat, and regulation of the mRNA levels of the leptin receptor subtypes in the hypothalamus during pregnancy and lactation. Biol Reproduct 62:698–703.

Gualillo O, Caminos JE, Blanco M, Garcia-Caballero T, Kojima M, Kangawa K, Dieguez C, Casanueva FF (2001) Ghrelin, a novel placental-derived hormone. Endocrinology 142:788–794.

Horvath TL, Diano S, Sotonyi P, Heiman M, Tschop M (2001) Ghrelin and the regulation of energy balance a hypothalamic perspective. Endocrinology 142:4163–4169.

Kalra SP, Dube MG, Pu S, Xu B, Horvath TL, Kalra PS (1999) Interacting appetite-regulating pathways in the hypothalamic regulation of body weight. Endocr Rev 20:68–100.

Kawai M, Yamaguchi M, Murakami T, Shima K, Murata Y, Kishi K (1997) The placenta is not the main source of leptin production in pregnant rat: gestational profile of leptin in plasma and adipose tissues. Biochem Biophys Res Commun 237:476–480.

Kojima M, Hosoda H, Date Y, Nakazato M, Matsuo M, Kangawa K (1999) Ghrelin is a growth hormone releasing acylated peptide from stomach. Nature 402:656–660.

Lage M, García-Mayor R, Tomé MA, Cordido F, Valle-Inclán F, Considine RV, Caro JF, Diéguez C, Casanueva FF (1999) Serum leptin levels in women throughout pregnancy and postpartum period and in women suffering spontaneous abortion. Clin Endocrinol 50:211–216.

Lee G, Proenca R, Montez JM, Carroll KM, Darvishzadeh JG, Lee JI, Friedman JM. (1996) Abnormal splicing of the leptin receptor in diabetic mice. Nature 379:632–635.

Lopez M, Seoane LM, Garcia MC, Lago F, Casanueva FF, Señaris RM, Dieguez C. (2000) Leptin regulation of prepro-orexin and orexin receptor mRNA levels in the hypothalamus. Biochem Biophys Res Commun 269:41–45.

Masuzaki H, Ogawa Y, Sagawa N, Hosoda K, Matsumoto T, Mise H, Nishimura H, Yoshimasa Y, Tanaka I, Mori T, Nakao K (1997) Nonadipose tissue production of leptin: leptin as a novel placenta-derived hormone in humans. Nature Med 3:1029–1033.

Murakami T, Yamashita T, Iida M, Kuwajima M, Shima I (1997) A short form of leptin receptor performs signal transduction. Biochem Biophys Res Commun 231:26–29.

Okada K, Ishii S, Minami S, Sugihara H, Shibasaki T, Wakabayashi I (1996) Intracerebroventricular administration of the growth hormone-releasing peptide KP-102 increases food intake in free-feeding rats. Endocrinology 137:5155–5158.

Qu D, Ludwig DS, Gammeltoft S, Piper M, Pelleymounter MA, Cullen MJ, Mathes WF, Przypek R, Kanarek R, Maratos-Flier E (1996) A role for melanin-concentrating hormone in the central regulation of feeding behaviour. Nature 380:243–247.

Richard D, Trayhurn P (1985) Energetic efficiency during pregnancy in mice fed ad libitum or pair-fed to the normal energy intake of unmated animals. J Nutr 115:593–600.

Sakurai T, Amemiya A, Ishii M, Matsuzaki I, Chemelli R, Tanaka H, Williams S, Richardson R, Kozlowski G, Wilson S, Arch J, Buckingham R, haynes A, carr S, Annan R, MacNutty D, Li W, Terret J, Elshourbagy N, Bergsma D, Yanagisawa M (1998) Orexin and orexin receptors: a family of hypothalamic neuropeptides and G-protein-coupled receptors that regulate feeding behaviour. Cell 92:573–585.

Señarís R, García-Caballero T, Casabiell X, Gallego R, Castro R, Considine RV, Diéguez C, Casanueva FF (1997) Synthesis of leptin in human placenta. Endocrinology 138:4501–4504.

Tartaglia LA (1997) The leptin receptor. J Biol Chem 272:6093–6096.

Tartaglia LA, Dembski M, Weng X, Deng N, Culpepper J, Devos R, Richards GJ, Campfield LA, Clark FT, Deeds J, Muir C, Sanker S, Moriarty A, Moore KJ, Smutko JS, Mays GG, Woolf EA, Monroe CA, Tepper RI (1995) Identification and expression cloning of a leptin receptor, OB-R. Cell 83:1263–1271.

Tomimatsu T, Yamaguchi M, Murakami T, Ogura K, Sakata M, Mitsuda N, Kanzaki T, Kurachi H, Irahara M, Miyake A, Shima K, Aono T, Murata Y (1997) Increase of mouse leptin production by adipose tissue after midpregnancy: gestational profile of serum leptin concentration. Biochem Biophys Res Commun 240:213–215.

Torsello A, Luoni M, Schweiger F, Grilli R, Guidi M, Bresciani E, Deghenghi R, Muller EE, Locatelli V (1998) Novel hexarelin analogs stimulate feeding in the rat through a mechanism not involving growth hormone release. Eur J Pharmacol 360:123–129.

Tschop M, Smiley DL, Helman ML (2000) Ghrelin induces adiposity in rodents. Nature 407:908–913.

White DW, Kuropatwinski KK, Devos R, Baumann H, Tartaglia LA (1997) Leptin receptor (OB-R) signaling. Cytoplasmic domain mutational analysis and evidence for receptor homo-oligomerization. J Biol Chem 272:4065–4071.

Willesen MG, Kristensen P, Romer J (1999) Co-localization of growth hormone secretagogue receptor and NPY mRNA in the arcuate nucleus of the rat. Neuroendocrinology 70:306–316.

Ghrelin: From GH Control to Feeding Behaviour and Sleep Regulatio

M.-T. Bluet-Pajot, V. Tolle, M.-H. Bassant, C. Kordon, P. Zizzari,
F. Poindessous-Jazat, C. Tomasetto[1], M. C. Rio[1], B. Estour[2], C. Foulon[3],
R. Dardennes[3], J. Epelbaum

Summary

Ghrelin, a 28-amino acid gastric peptide with a n-octanoylation on Ser 3, has recently been identified as an endogenous ligand of the growth hormone secretagogue receptor (GHS-R). In parallel a cDNA encoding a protein which shares sequence similarities with prepromotilin was isolated from a mouse stomach library and its putative product was named prepromotilin-related peptide (ppMTLRP). Mouse and rat ppMTLRP sequences are identical and show 89 % identity with human ghrelin. By analogy with promotilin, cleavage of proMTLRP into an 18-amino acid endogenous processed peptide was assumed on the basis of a conserved dibasic motif in position 19–20 of ghrelin sequence. In freely moving animals, both rat and human ghrelin stimulated GH release and human ghrelin 18 was ineffective, whereas in vitro, on superfused pituitaries, the three peptides stimulated GH release to the same extent. Activation of somatostatin (SRIF) release by ether stress did not modify GH response to ghrelin in vivo and ghrelin blunted 25 mM K+-induced-SRIF release from perifused hypothalami in vitro. This finding suggests that ghrelin action on GH secretion is mediated, at least partially, through functional antagonism of somatostatin.

Ghrelin is not only effective on GH secretion but also increases gastrointestinal motility and displays orexigenic effects. This multiplicity of effects is in keeping with the pattern of GHS-R expression on hypothalamic Neuropeptide Y, SRIF and GHRH neurons. However, the relationships between endogenous ghrelin and GH secretions and feeding and sleep patterns remained to be investigated. In freely moving adult male rats, repeated administration of ghrelin at 3 to 4-h intervals (one during light-on and two during light-off periods) immediately increased GH release feeding activity and wakefulness while it decreased sleep duration. However, on the total duration of the sampling period (nine hours), only the stimulation of GH secretion and the inhibition of REM sleep were maintained. Endogenous plasma ghrelin levels exhibited pulsatile variations of smaller amplitude and regularity as compared to those of GH. The circulating levels of the two hormones were not strictly correlated, although mean interpeak intervals and pulse frequencies were close. In contrast, ghrelin pulse variations were correlated with food intake episodes in the light-off period and plasma ghrelin concentrations

INSERM U549 and [1]CMME, IFR Broca Ste-Anne, 2 ter rue d'Alésia, 75014 Paris, [3]IGBMC, CNRS/INSERM U184/ULP, Illkirch and [2]Hôpital Bellevue St Etienne, France

Kordon et al.
Brain Somatic Cross-Talk and the
Central Control of Metabolism
© Springer-Verlag Berlin Heidelberg 2002

decreased by 26 % in the 20 minutes following the end of the food intake periods. A positive correlation between ghrelin levels and active wake was found during the first three hours of the light-off period only. Since ghrelin secretion appeared to be directly related to feeding behaviour, we assessed its plasma levels in anorexia nervosa patients before and after renutrition in comparison with constitutionally thin subjects. Morning fasting plasma ghrelin was doubled in anorexia nervosa patients as compared to age-matched, constitutionally thin women, and it returned to normal values in patients after renutrition.

In summary, ghrelin, which was discovered as a GH-secreting factor from the stomach, appears to also be related to the control of feeding behaviour. Whether ghrelin per se or through its indirect effects on feeding (and all attendant metabolic sequelae) acts on sleep remains to be determined.

Introduction

Ghrelin, a 28-amino acid acylated peptide purified from the stomach (Fig. 1A), is an endogenous ligand for the growth hormone secretagogue receptor (GHS-R; Kojima et al. 1999) and exhibits structural resemblance to motilin, a 22-amino acid peptide involved in the regulation of interdigestive motility (Tomasetto et al. 2000). A few ghrelin-immunoreactive neurons have been visualized in the hypothalamus in arcuate parvocellular neurons (Kojima et al. 1999) and in paraventricular and supraoptic magnocellular neurons (Kagotani et al. 2001), but the bulk of the peptide expression is restricted to the stomach (Nass et al. 2001) and circulating ghrelin levels are considerably reduced in gastrectomized patients (Ariyasu et al. 2001).

In rodents, ghrelin has recently been shown to not only stimulate growth hormone (GH) secretion (Seoane et al. 2000; Tolle et al. 2001) but also exert gastroprokinetic (Masuda et al. 2000), orexigenic and adipogenic effects (Asakawa et al. 2001a; Tschop et al. 2000; Wren et al. 2000). Effects on GH secretion (Arvat et al. 2000; Nagaya et al. 2001; Peino et al. 2000; Takaya et al. 2000) and feeding behaviour (Toshinai et al. 2001; Tschop et al. 2001a, b; Wren et al. 2001) are also observed in the human species. As recently reviewed, the dual action on GH secretion, and food intake as well as the dual localization of ghrelin and its receptors in hypothalamus and stomach immediately raised the question of the interdependency of these actions (Bowers 2001). Many studies have linked nutrition and episodic GH secretion although these relationships vary from species to species, with undernutrition reducing GH pulsatility in the rat while the converse is true in humans (Robinson and Hindmarsh 1999). One common property of feeding behaviour and GH secretion is their rhythmicity. The pulsatile mode of GH secretion depends primarily on the coordinate actions of hypothalamic growth hormone releasing hormone (GHRH) and somatostatin (SRIF) release from median eminence terminals, but multiple intra- and extra-pituitary regulatory signals and diurnally varying neuronal inputs related to the sleep-wake pattern are also involved (Giustina and Veldhuis 1998; Van Cauter and Copinschi 2000). In return, feeding behaviour is also dependent on the interaction of regulatory signals, including sleep-wake patterns, and diurnally neuronal inputs on a complex array of hypothalamic peptidergic neurons (Stanley et al. 1986). It was therefore of interest to assess the importance of ghrelin in these interactions.

In vivo and in vitro effects of ghrelin/motilin related peptide on GH and somatostatin secretion in the rat.

In freely moving rats ghrelin stimulated GH release (Fig. 1) but did not affect plasma prolactin, ACTH or leptin levels (data not shown). In contrast, the shorter form, ghrelin18, and non-octanoylated ghrelin were ineffective. In vitro, ghrelin stimulated GH release from superfused pituitaries in a dose-dependent manner but the amplitude of the effect was much lower than in vivo. In vitro GH responses to ghrelin or to the shorter form ghrelin18 (this latter in contrast to in vivo data) were comparable (Fig. 1C). Non-octanoylated ghrelin was ineffective in vitro as already observed in vivo.

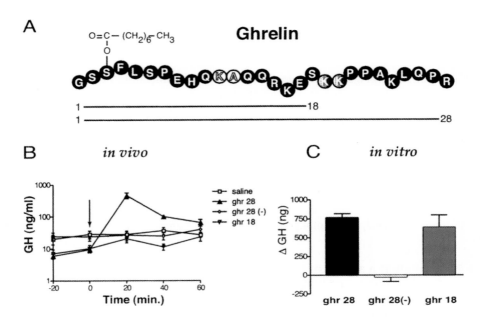

Fig. 1. Structure and effects of ghrelin peptides on GH release in vivo and in vitro. A. Ghrelin (ghr), identified as an endogenous ligand of the growth hormone secretagogue receptor (GHS-R) is a 28-amino acid gastric peptide N-octanoylated on Ser 3 (ghr 28). Parallely, a cDNA encoding a protein with 89% identity with human ghrelin and 33% similarities with prepromotilin was isolated from a mouse stomach library. By analogy with promotilin, cleavage of proghr into an 18-amino acid endogenous processed peptide (ghr 18) was assumed on the basis of a conserved dibasic motif in position 19–20 of its sequence. B. In freely moving, young adult male rats, ghr28 stimulates GH release whereas non-octanoylated ghr 28(–) and ghr18 are ineffective. C. In vitro, on superfused rat pituitaries, ghr 28 and ghr 18 stimulate GH release equally whereas ghr 28(–) remains ineffective.

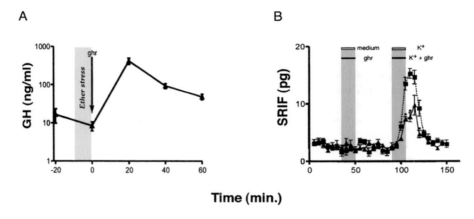

Fig. 2. Functional antagonism of SRIF by ghrelin in vivo and in vitro. **A.** The ether stress-in-duced inhibition of GH secretion in vivo (likely mediated through SRIF release) does not inter-fere with the GH-releasing effects of ghrelin. **B.** Ghr directly inhibits K^+ depolarization-induced SRIF release from superfused rat hypothalamus.

Under stressful conditions known to stimulate hypothalamic SRIF release (i.e., within 10 minutes of exposure to ether), the amplitude of ghrelin-induced GH re-lease was comparable to that obtained in non-anaesthetized animals (Fig. 2A). When tested on perifused hypothalamic tissue, ghrelin significantly inhibited 25 mM K+ depolarization-induced SRIF release (Fig. 2B).

Thus ghrelin effects on GH are likely to be mediated, at least in part, through functional antagonism of SRIF release (see also Drisko et al. 1999) in accordance with the partial colocalization of GHS-R mRNA expression on SRIF and GHRH hypothalamic neurons (Willesen et al. 1999; see also Tannenbaum et al., this vol-ume). GHS-R mRNA expression on a greater proportion of Neuropeptide Y in-terneurons is likely to be important for the effect of ghrelin on feeding behaviour.

Effect of ghrelin administration on growth hormone secretion, feeding behaviour and states of arousal in rats

Administration of ghrelin at 1020 hours (light period), 1420 hours and 1720 hours (dark period) always resulted in a rapid modification of GH release, feed-ing behaviour and sleep-wake pattern during the 30 minutes following each in-jection (Fig. 3, upper panels). GH secretion was strongly stimulated and food in-take always lasted longer in ghrelin-treated than in saline-injected rats. During the 30 minutes after ghrelin injection, in the light-on and the beginning of the light-off period, wakefulness was increased and slow wave and REM sleep de-creased. However, during the nine-hour observation period (Fig. 3, lower panels), the total amount of GH released was almost doubled in treated animals where as food intake duration and the quantity of food ingested were not different. Total

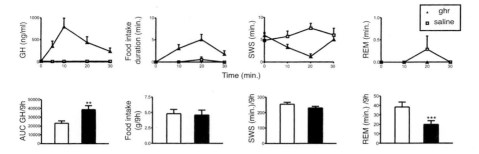

Fig. 3. Comparison of acute and long-term ghrelin effects on GH secretion, food intake and sleep wake patterns in adult rats. **Upper panels.** Acute (30 minutes after the injection) effects of ghr (10 µg/rat) on GH plasma levels, food intake duration, slow wave sleep (SWS) and paradoxical sleep (REM) durations. **Lower panels.** Long-term effects on the nine-hour sampling period (from 1000 to 1900 hours; ghr injections at 1020, 1420 and 1720 hours).

wakefulness and SWS durations were unchanged but REM sleep was significantly decreased. The mean number of REM sequences remained unchanged, whereas the mean duration of each sequence was markedly decreased (56 ± 8 vs 99 ± 9 sec, P< 0.01).

At this stage, it remained to be determined if endogenous plasma ghrelin secretion was pulsatile and what its relationships to GH secretion, feeding behaviour and sleep-wake patterns were.

Relationships between endogenous plasma ghrelin levels, growth hormone secretion, feeding behaviour and states of arousal.

In young freely moving adult male rats, plasma ghrelin levels (Fig. 4A), measured every 20 minutes over nine hours, exhibited pulsatile variations of modest amplitude when compared to those of GH secretion (Fig. 4B). No direct correlation between GH and ghrelin secretory patterns was found. Food intake episodes (Fig. 4C) were more regular than ghrelin pulsatile variations but not significantly different from those of GH. A positive correlation between AUC ghrelin and duration of active wake (Fig. 4D) occurred during the first three hours of the dark period (r = 0.769; p = 0.0257). Cross-ApEn analysis revealed that GH and food intake and ghrelin and food intake rhythms were more synchronized than GH and ghrelin secretory patterns (Fig. 4E).

The direct relationship between endogenous ghrelin plasma levels and food intake in rats as well as in humans (Cummings et al. 2001) led us to assess this parameter in human subjects with a disturbance in feeding behaviour, namely Anorexia Nervosa patients.

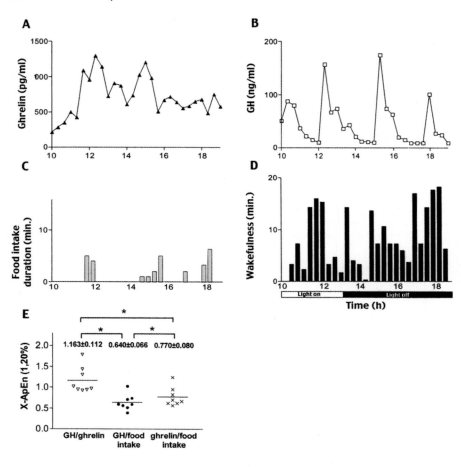

Fig. 4. Representative profiles of ghrelin and GH secretion, food intake episodes, and wakefulness showing the temporal relationships beteween these parameters. **A.** Ghrelin. **B.** GH. **C.** Food intake. **D.** Wakefulness. **E.** CrossApen (X-ApEn) indicates a higher synchrony of ghr secretion and food intake than ghr and GH secretion.

Circulating ghrelin in Anorexia Nervosa patients and constitutionally thin women

Anorexia Nervosa is a syndrome generally seen in young women under 25 which combines weight loss, ammenorhea and behavioral changes. These endocrine and psychological changes appear to be reversible with weight gain. It is generally supposed that a unique abnormality, probably of hypothalamic origin, is involved in this adaptation to the starvation state. In the same age range as Anorexia Nervosa, a non-pathologic state exists that has been denominated constitutional thinness (Biadi et al. 2001). These young women present with very low body mass indexes (BMI <16.5), no ammenorhea and no behavioral changes. The neuroen-docrine mechanisms regulating GH secretion are strongly dependent on nutritional states. In humans, fasting stimulates GH release, and Anorexia Nervosa patients show elevated basal GH in the presence of low IGF-1 levels (Stoving et al.

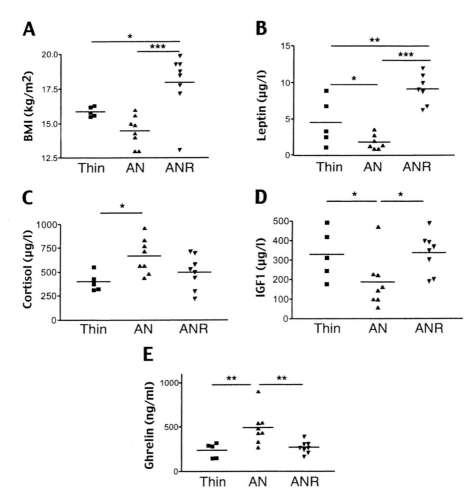

Fig. 5. Comparison of fasting endocrine parameters in constitutionally thin subjects and Anorexia Nervosa patients before and after renutrition. **A.** Body mass indexs (BMI) are similar in constitutionally thin subjects (Thin) and Anorexia Nervosa (AN) patients. They are significantly increased in patients following renutrition (ANR). **B.** Leptin levels are lower in AN as compared to Thin and are elevated in ANR. **C.** Cortisol levels are elevated in AN and return to Thin values in ANR. **D.** IGF-I levels are lower in AN as compared to Thin and return to normal values after renutrition. **E.** Ghrelin levels are significantly elevated in AN as compared to Thin and return to normal values after renutrition.

Fig. 6. Schematic representation of ghrelin interactions in the neuroendocrine control of GH secretion and feeding behaviour. Circulating ghrelin, originating essentially from the stomach, acts primarily on intrahypothalamic GHS-receptors located on arcuate GHRH and Neuropeptide Y (NPY) neurons, the former being more implicated in the control of GH secretion and the latter in feeding behaviour. Ghrelin also acts directly on pituitary somatotrophs to moderately stimulate GH secretion. The mechanisms by which ghrelin antagonizes SRIF release and action on GH secretion remain elusive but appears mediated through sst2 SRIF receptors (Zheng et al. 1997). Thus, ghrelin can be considered as a third peripheral hormone which, together with IGF-I and leptin, is involved in the control of intrahypothalamic neuroendocrine neuronal networks. ARC, arcuate nucleus; PeV, periventricular area.

⟶

1999). However, the mechanisms subserving these changes remain unclear. As shown on Figure 5, Anorexia Nervosa patients displayed BMI similar to constitutionally thin women, whereas their plasma leptin and IGF-1 levels were decreased and their cortisol levels were increased. After Anorexia Nervosa renutrition, BMI and plasma leptin levels were increased and IGF-I and cortisol levels returned to control values. The morning fasting plasma ghrelin level was 238 ± 37 ng/L (n=5) in young, constitutionally thin women. It reached 491 ± 68 (n=8) in Anorexia Nervosa patients ($p<0.05$) and returned to 269 ± 54 (n=8) in patients after renutrition (see also Ariyasu et al. 2001; Wren et al. 2001). On the other hand, circulating ghrelin levels are decreased in human obesity (Tschop et al. 2001a), and a single base mutation in the preproghrelin gene has been reported in this latter disease (Ukkola et al. 2001).

Acknowledgments

This work was supported by INSERM and its ATC Nutrition.

Conclusion

Two years after its discovery, the action of ghrelin as a new GH-secretagogue, both at the pituitary and hypothalamic levels, has been confirmed in most species tested so far. In addition, ghrelin appears to be involved in the regulation of food intake (see Fig. 6). However, the demonstration that endogenous ghrelin is involved in the regulation of GH pulsatility has not yet been made. In contrast, both in humans and rats a direct relationship exists between circulating ghrelin concentrations and food intake episodes. The relationships between this last function and the fact that ghrelin appears able to modify sleep-wake patterns and anxiety (Asakawa et al. 2001b) warrant further investigations.

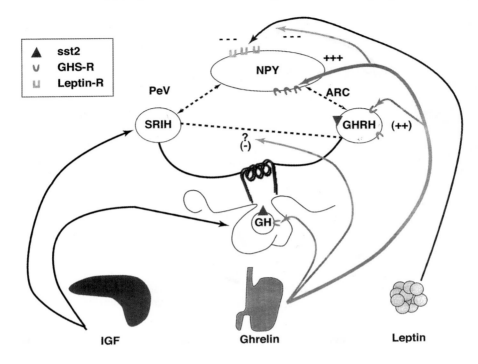

References

Ariyasu H, Takaya K, Tagami T, Ogawa Y, Hosoda H, Akamizu T, Suda M, Koh T, Natsui K, Toyooka S, Shirakami G, Usui T, Shimatsu A, Doi K, Hosoda H, Kojima M, Kangawa K, Nakao K (2001) Stomach is a major source of circulating ghrelin, and feeding state determines plasma ghrelin-like immunoreactivity levels in humans. J Clin Endocrinol Metab 86:4753–4758

Arvat E, Di Vito L, Broglio F, Papotti M, Muccioli G, Dieguez C, Casanueva FF, Deghenghi R, Camanni F, Ghigo E (2000) Preliminary evidence that Ghrelin, the natural GH secretagogue (GHS)-receptor ligand, strongly stimulates GH secretion in humans. J Endocrinol Investi 23:493–495

Asakawa A, Inui A, Kaga T, Yuzuriha H, Nagata T, Ueno N, Makino S, Fujimiya M, Niijima A, Fujino MA, Kasuga M (2001a) Ghrelin is an appetite-stimulatory signal from stomach with structural resemblance to motilin. Gastroenterology 120:337–345

Asakawa A, Inui A, Kaga T, Yuzuriha H, Nagata T, Fujimiya M, Katsuura G, Makino S, Fujino MA, Kasuga M (2001b) A role of ghrelin in neuroendocrine and behavioral responses to stress in mice. Neuroendocrinology 74:143–147

Biadi O, Rossini R, Musumeci G, Frediani L, Masullo M, Ramacciotti C, Dellosso L, Paoli R, Mariotti R, Cassano G, Mariani M (2001) Cardiopulmonary exercise test in young women affected by anorexia nervosa. Ital Heart J 2(6):462–467.

Bowers CY (2001) Unnatural growth hormone-releasing peptide begets natural ghrelin. J Clin Endocrinol Metab 86:1464–1469.

Cummings D, Purnell J, Frayo R, Schmidova K, BEW, Weigle D (2001) A prandial rise in plasma ghrelin levels suggests a role in meal initiation in humans. Diabetes 50(8):1714–1719

Drisko J, Faidley T, Zhang D, McDonald T, Nicolich S, Hora D, Cunningham P, Li C, Rickes E, McNamara L, Chang C, Smith R, Hickey G (1999) Administration of a nonpeptidyl growth hormone secretagogue, L-163, 255, changes somatostatin pattern, but has no effect on patterns of growth hormone-releasing factor in the hypophyseal-portal circulation of the conscious pig. Proc Soc Exp Biol Med 222(1):70–77

Giustina A, Veldhuis JD (1998) Pathophysiology of the neuroregulation of growth hormone secretion in experimental animals and the human. Endocr Rev 19:717–797.

Kagotani Y, Sakata I, Yamazaki M, Nakamuea K, Hayashi Y, Kangawa K, Sakai T (2001) Localization of ghrelin immunopositive cells in the rat hypothalamus and gastrointestinal tract. Proc 83rd Meeting of the endocrine society, Denver, CO, 2001, 337.

Kojima M, Hosoda H, Date Y, Nakazato M, Matsuo H, Kangawa K (1999) Ghrelin is a growth-hormone-releasing acylated peptide from stomach. Nature 402:656–660

Masuda Y, Tanaka T, Inomata N, Ohnuma N, Tanaka S, Itoh Z, Hosoda H, Kojima M, Kangawa K (2000) Ghrelin stimulates gastric acid secretion and motility in rats. Biochem Biophys Res Commun 276:905–908.

Nagaya N, Kojima M, Uematsu M, Yamagishi M, Hosoda H, Oya H, Hayashi Y, Kangawa K (2001) Hemodynamic and hormonal effects of human ghrelin in healthy volunteers. Am J Physiol Regul Integr Comp Physiol 280:R1483–1487.

Nass R, Hellmann P, Gaylinn B, Thorner MO (2001) Measurement of ghrelin mRNA in stomach, pituitary and hypothalamus of young adult rats. Proc 83rd Meeting of the endocrine society, Denver, CO, 2001, 327.

Peino R, Baldelli R, Rodriguez-Garcia J, Rodriguez-Segade S, Kojima M, Kangawa K, Arvat E, Ghigo E, Dieguez C, Casanueva FF (2000) Ghrelin-induced growth hormone secretion in humans. Eur J Endocrinol 143:R11–R14

Robinson I.C.A.F. & Hindmarsh P.C. (1999) The Growth Hormone secretory pattern and statural growth. in The Endocrine System Vol V : Hormonal control of Growth, J.L. Kostyo volume ed., H. M. Goodman, series ed. Oxford University Press (New York, Oxford), pp 330–396.

Seoane LM, Tovar S, Baldelli R, Arvat E, Ghigo E, Casanueva FF, Dieguez C (2000) Ghrelin elicits a marked stimulatory effect on GH secretion in freely-moving rats. Eur J Endocrinol 143:R007–R009

Stanley BG, Kyrkouli SE, Lampert S, Leibowitz SF (1986) Neuropeptide Y chronically injected into the hypothalamus: a powerful neurochemical inducer of hyperphagia and obesity. Peptides 7:1189–1192.

Stoving R, Veldhuis J, Flyvbjerg A, Vinten J, Hangaard J, Koldkjaer O, Kristiansen J, Hagen C (1999) Jointly amplified basal and pulsatile growth hormone (GH) secretion and increased process irregularity in women with anorexia nervosa: indirect evidence for disruption of feedback regulation within the GH-insulin-like growth factor I axis. J Clin Endocrinol Metab 84(6):2056–2063

Takaya K, Ariyasu H, Kanamoto N, Iwakura H, Yoshimoto A, Harada M, Mori K, Komatsu Y, Usui T, Shimatsu A, Ogawa Y, Hosoda K, Akamizu T, Kojima M, Kangawa K, Nakao K (2000) Ghrelin strongly stimulates growth hormone (GH) release in humans. J Clin Endocrinol Metab 85:4908–4911

Tolle V, Zizzari P, Tomasetto C, Rio MC, Epelbaum J, Bluet-Pajot MT (2001) In vivo and in vitro effects of ghrelin/motilin-related peptide on growth hormone secretion in the rat. Neuroendocrinology 73:54–61.

Tomasetto C, Karam SM, Ribieras S, Masson R, Lefebvre O, Staub A, Alexander G, Chenard MP, Rio MC (2000) Identification and characterization of a novel gastric peptide hormone: the motilin-related peptide. Gastroenterology 119:395–405.

Toshinai K, Mondal MS, Nakazato M, Date Y, Murakami N, Kojima M, Kangawa K, Matsukura S (2001) Upregulation of Ghrelin expression in the stomach upon fasting, insulin-induced hypoglycemia, and leptin administration. Biochem Biophys Res Commun 281:1220–1225.

Tschop M, Smiley DL, Heiman ML (2000) Ghrelin induces adiposity in rodents. Nature 407:908–913

Tschop M, Weyer C, Tataranni PA, Devanarayan V, Ravussin E, Heiman ML (2001a) Circulating ghrelin levels are decreased in human obesity. Diabetes 50:707–709.

Tschop M, Wawarta R, Riepl RL, Friedrich S, Bidlingmaier M, Landgraf R, Folwaczny C (2001b) Post-prandial decrease of circulating human ghrelin levels. J Endocrinol Invest 24:RC19–21.

Ukkola O, Ravussin E, Jacobson P, Snyder E, Chagnon M, Sjostrom L, Bouchard C (2001) Mutations in the preproghrelin/ghrelin gene associated with obesity in humans. J Clin Endocrinol Metab 86(8):3996–3999

Van Cauter E, Copinschi G (2000) Interrelationships between growth hormone and sleep. Growth Hormone Igf Res 10:57–62

Willesen M, Kristensen P, Romer J (1999) Co-localization of growth hormone secretagogue receptor and NPY mRNA in the arcuate nucleus of the rat. Neuroendocrinology 70(5):306–316

Wren AM, Small CJ, Ward HL, Murphy KG, Dakin CL, Taheri S, Kennedy AR, Roberts GH, Morgan DGA, Ghatei MA, Bloom SR (2000) The novel hypothalamic peptide ghrelin stimulates food intake and growth hormone secretion. Endocrinology 141:4325–4328

Wren AM, Seal LJ, Cohen MA, Brynes AE, Frost GS, Murphy KG, Dhillo WS, Ghatei MA, Bloom SR (2001) Ghrelin enhances appetite and increases food Intake in humans. J Clin Endocrinol Metab 86:5992

Zheng H, Bailey A, Jiang MH, Honda K, Chen HY, Trumbauer ME, van der Ploeg LHT, Schaeffer JM, Leng G, Smith RG (1997) Somatostatin receptor subtype 2 knock out mice are refractory to growth hormone negative feedback on arcuate neurons. Mol Endocrinol 11:1709–1717

Effect of Leptin on Fatless Mice

I. Shimomura[1]

Summary

Generalized lipodystrophy (GL) is a disorder characterized by a paucity of adipose (fat) tissue that is accompanied by a severe resistance to insulin, leading to hyperinsulinemia, hyperglycemia, and enlarged fatty liver. Our laboratory have developed a mouse model that mimics these features of generalized lipodystrophy: the syndrome occurs in transgenic mice expressing a truncated version of a nuclear protein known as nSREBP-1c (sterol-regulatory-element-binding protein-1c) under the control of the adipose-specific aP2 enhancer. Adipose tissue from these mice was markedly deficient in mRNAs encoding several fat-specific proteins, including leptin, a fat-derived hormone that regulates food intake and energy metabolism. We revealed that insulin resistance in lipodystrophic mice can be overcome by a continuous systemic infusion of recombinant leptin, an effect that is not mimicked by chronic food restriction. These results support the idea that leptin modulates insulin sensitivity and glucose disposal independently of its effect on food intake. As humans with generalized lipodystrophy have extremely low levels of plasma leptin, clinical trials of leptin treatment in these patients are warranted.

In lipodystrophic mice, leptin deficiency leads to hyperglycemia, hyperinsulinemia, and insulin resistance. In this condition, the liver overproduces glucose as a result of resistance to the normal action of insulin in repressing mRNAs for gluconeogenic enzymes. We found that chronic hyperinsulinemia downregulates the mRNA for IRS-2, an essential component in the insulin signaling in liver, thereby producing insulin resistance. Despite IRS-2 deficiency, insulin continues to stimulate production of SREBP-1c, a transcriptional factor that activates fatty acid synthesis. The combination of insulin resistance (inappropriate gluconeogenesis) and insulin sensitivity (elevated lipogenesis) establishes a vicious cycle that aggravates hyperinsulinemia and insulin resistance in lipodystrophy.

The results obtained from mice were successfully applied to human disease. Leptin administration was reported to improve insulin resistance syndrome, including diabetes, hyperlipidemia and fatty liver in patients with generalized lipodystrophy.

[1]Department of Frontier Bioscience Graduate School of Frontier Bioscience, Osaka University and Department of Medicine and Pathophysiology Graduate School of Medicine, Osaka University 2-2 Yamadaoka, Suita, Osaka 565-0871, Japan

Kordon et al.
Brain Somatic Cross-Talk and the
Central Control of Metabolism
© Springer-Verlag Berlin Heidelberg 2002

Physiological significance
of Sterol regulatory element-binding proteins (SREBPs)

Sterol regulatory element-binding proteins (SREBPs) are transcription factors that activate transcription of multiple genes encoding enzymes of cholesterol and fatty acid synthesis in liver and other tissues (Brown and Goldstein 1997). Over-production of dominant active SREBPs in livers of transgenic mice resulted in massive hepatic accumulation of lipids (Horton et al. 1998; Horton and Shimomura 1999; Shimano et al. 1996, 1997). This observation demonstrated that over-activity of SREBPs could underlie lipid accumulation in liver in pathologic states. This conclusion was supported by data from several laboratories (Foretz et al. 1999; Shimomura et al. 1999a,b), including our own, which showed that insulin increases the nuclear content of one isoform of SREBP (SREBP-1c) in liver cells, and that this appears to constitute the mechanism by which insulin stimulates hepatic lipid synthesis.

SREBPs belong to the basic-helix-loop-helix-leucine zipper family of transcription factors (Brown and Goldstein 1997). They are synthesized as ≈1150 amino acid precursors bound to the endoplasmic reticulum (ER). To become active, the NH_2-terminal segment of SREBPs, called the nuclear form, is released from the membrane by a two-step cleavage process. When cells require sterols and fatty acids, SREBPs are cleaved and translocate to the nucleus to activate the transcription of target genes. Three SREBP isoforms are known. SREBP-1a and -1c are derived from a single gene through the use of alternative transcription start sites that produce alternate forms of exon 1 (Hua et al. 1995; Yokoyama et al. 1993). The third SREBP isoform, SREBP-2, is derived from a separate gene (Hua et al. 1993). In most animal tissues, including liver and adipose tissue, SREBP-1c is the predominant SREBP-1 isoform (Shimomura et al. 1997a,b). The SREBP isoforms have different transcriptional activation properties. SREBP-1a and -1c isoforms preferentially activate genes involved in the synthesis of fatty acids and triglycerides, whereas SREBP-2 preferentially activates genes involved in cholesterol biosynthesis (Horton et al 1998; Horton and Shimomura 1999).

aP2-SREBP-1c transgenic mice: a mouse model
for human generalized lipodystrophy

The SREBP-1c isoform has been implicated in adipose differentiation. Rat SREBP-1c cDNA was isolated independently by Tontonoz et al. (1993). When the SREBP-1c protein was expressed in 3T3-L1 adipocytes, differentiation was enhanced and, hence, the protein was named adipocyte determination and differentiation factor-1 (ADD1) (Tortonoz et al. 1993; Kim and Spiegelman 1996; Kim et al. 1998). When 3T3-L1 cells are stimulated to differentiate, SREBP-1 mRNA rises markedly. Our laboratory established a RNase protection assay to discriminate between the SREBP-1a and -1c isoforms and found that only the mRNA for SREBP-1a increased (Shimomura et al. 1997b). To further explore the in vivo roles of the SREBP-1 isoforms in adipose tissue, our laboratory generated transgenic mice that overexpress the constitutively active nuclear from of SREBP-1c in adipose tissues using the adipocyte-specific aP2 promoter (Shimomura et al. 1998). The surprising result was that the overexpression did not enhance adipocyte differentiation. Indeed, it blocked differentiation of both white and brown adipose tissue, producing a syndrome analogous to congenital generalized lipodystrophy in humans.

The transgenic mice that overexpress the nuclear form of SREBP-1c exclusively in adipose tissue exhibit the following features of congenital generalized lipodystrophy (CGL) (Seip and Trygstad 1996): 1) disordered adipocyte differentiation resulting in marked reduction in the amount of adipose tissue; 2) marked insulin resistance manifested by hyperglycemia in the face of a 50- to 200-fold elevation in plasma insulin; and 3) fatty liver and elevated plasma triglycerides.

Leptin treatment of lipodystrophy

The lipodystrophic mice had low plasma leptin levels, presumably due to the disturbed adipose tissue differentiation. Leptin is a fat-derived hormone that regulates food intake and energy metabolism (Friedman and Halaas 1998). As a result of leptin deficiency, the lipodystrophic mice overeat and become markedly hyperglycemic and insulin resistant (Shimomura et al. 1998). The livers of the lipodystrophic mice are engorged with triglyceride. Our laboratory found that hepatic triglyceride accumulation was associated with elevated SREBP-1c mRNA and protein levels (Shimomura et al 1999a). In addition, the mRNAs for genes involved in lipogenesis were coordinately increased. Remarkably, our laboratory showed that the abnormalities in liver and plasma of the lipodystrophic mice, like those of *ob/ob* mice, were reversed by administration of recombinant leptin (Shimomura et al. 1999c). Restoration of physiologic leptin levels led to a significant decline in plasma insulin and glucose levels, and the excess hepatic triglyceride largely disappeared. In contrast, the chronic restriction of food intake did not normalize glucose and lipid homeostasis.

Pathophysiology underlying lipodystrophy: coexistence of insulin resistance and insulin sensitivity in livers of lipodystrophic and ob/ob mice

The livers of lipodystrophic and *ob/ob* mice overproduce glucose despite the presence of hyperinsulinemia and hyperglycemia. Normally, insulin represses the mRNAs for gluconeogenic enzymes. This action of insulin is absent in livers of insulin-resistant mice. In contrast, hyperinsulinemia continues to activate fatty acid biosynthesis resulting in hepatic triglyceride accumulation. To explain these phenomena, Our laboratory found alterations of the mRNAs encoding two crucial proteins in these livers (Shimomura et al. 2000). One is IRS-2, an essential component of the insulin-signaling pathway in the liver. IRS-2 mRNA was markedly decreased, potentially explaining the insulin resistance. In contrast, the mRNA encoding SREBP-1c was elevated, an event that may explain the continued activity of insulin to stimulate lipid synthesis despite the other manifestation of insulin resistance.

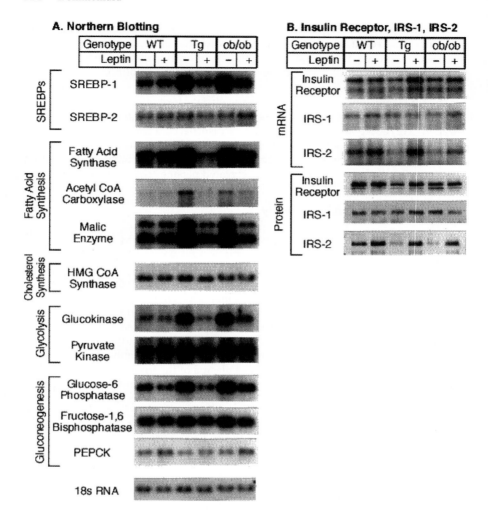

Fig. 1. Changes in mRNA and protein levels in livers of wild-type (WT), transgenic lipodys-trophic (Tg), and *ob/ob* mice treated with or without leptin. **A)** Northern blot analysis of mRNAs associated with specific metabolic pathways. **B)** Northern blot and immunoblot analysis of insulin receptor, IRS-1, and IRS-2. Data from Shimomura et al. (2000)

Insulin sensitivity (increased lipogenesis)

It has long been known that hepatic lipogenesis is activated by insulin (Hillgart-ner et al. 1995; Waters and Ntambi 1994). This activation is mediated by post-transcriptional mechanisms as well as by an insulin-mediated increase in the transcription of genes encoding key lipogenic enzymes, such as fatty acid synthetase (FAS) and acetyl-CoA carboxylase (ACC). The mRNAs encoding these proteins were increased in the hyperinsulinemic lipodystrophic and *ob/ob* mice (Shimomura et al. 1999a), indicating a normal response to insulin. Figure 1A compares the levels of various mRNAs in livers of wild-type, lipodystrophic, and *ob/ob* mice treated with saline or with leptin. The mRNA for SREBP-1 was significantly elevated in livers of both hyperinsulinemic mouse models, and it was normalized when plasma insulin fell as a result of leptin treatment. The changes measured in SREBP-1 mRNA were attributed solely to the mRNA for the SREBP-1c isoform, as measured by RNase protection assay. The mRNAs for the SREBP-1c target genes – acetyl CoA carboxylase, fatty acid synthetase, and malic enzyme (lipogenesis), and glucokinase and pyruvate (enzymes of glycolysis) – rose and fell in parallel with the SREBP-1c mRNA. These data indicate that the genes encoding glycolytic and lipogenic enzymes responded appropriately to the elevated insulin levels in the lipodystrophic and *ob/ob* mice. Recently, our laboratory and others have shown that insulin's induction of glycolytic and lipogenic enzymes in liver is mediated by an increase in the SREBP-1c mRNA and a subsequent increase in the nuclear SREBP-1c protein (Foretz et al. 1999; Shimomura et al. 1999a,b). These data suggest that the pathway linking the insulin receptor and SREBP-1c regulation is intact in hyperinsulinemic animals.

Insulin resistance

Insulin resistance in the livers of hyperinsulinemic mice was manifested by an elevation of the mRNAs for the gluconeogenic enzymes glucose-6-phosphatase, fructose-1,6-bisphosphatase and phosphoenolpyruvate carboxykinase (PEPCK; Fig. 1A). If insulin had been acting normally, these mRNAs should have been severely reduced in hyperinsulinemic mice (Hall and Granner 1996; O'Brien and Granner 1996). The mRNAs encoding the insulin receptor and IRS-1 were unchanged in livers of these mice. In contrast, IRS-2 mRNA and protein levels were markedly reduced in livers, and leptin infusion raised the IRS-2 mRNA and protein levels to normal in these mice (Fig. 1B; Shimomura et al. 2000).

The fall in IRS-2 mRNA and protein in the insulin-resistant mice is a potentially significant finding because IRS-2 is a major component of the insulin-signaling pathway. This pathway is initiated by insulin binding, which activates the insulin receptor tyrosine kinase, which in turn polyphosphorylates insulin receptor substrate-1 (IRS-1) and IRS-2 (Virkamaki et al. 1999). Phosphorylated tyrosines on IRS-1 and IRS-2 activate phosphoinositide 3-kinase (PI3-kinase), which leads to phosphorylation of Akt. Active Akt phosphorylates insulin-regulated enzymes, thereby mediating many of the post-transcriptional effects of insulin, including the suppression of gluconeogenesis (Virkamaki et al. 1999). To determine whether the reduction in IRS-2 interfered with insulin signaling, I measured the ability of a high dose of insulin to increase IRS-associated PI3-kinase and to enforce phosphorylation of Akt (Fig. 2). Our laboratory injected 5 units of insulin or PBS intraportally to wild-type and lipodystrophic mice (Shimomura et al. 2000). The livers were excised 1 min after the injection. As shown in Figure 1, IRS-2 protein was selectively reduced in the transgenic livers whereas the amount of IRS-1 protein was not altered (Fig. 2A). The amount of total Akt was normal in lipodystrophic livers. Our laboratory did not see an increase of phospho-Akt in the livers of the lipodystrophic mice at time 0, despite the high levels of circulating insulin. Insulin increased the amount of phospho-Akt in the wild-type liver. In contrast, there was no increase in phosphorylation of Akt in the lipodystrophic liver. This finding paralleled the IRS-2-associated PI3-kinase activity (Fig. 2B; unpublished observation; Shimomura, I. et al). The acute insulin administration caused a large increase in PI3-kinase activity bound to IRS-1 (lanes 1 and 2) and IRS-2 (lanes 5 and 6) in wild-type mice. The amount of PI3-kinase associated with IRS-1 was higher in lipodystrophic livers at baseline than controls (lanes 1 and 3) but the amount associated with IRS-2 was significantly reduced (lanes 5 and 7). There was a further increase in IRS-1 associated PI3-kinase when insulin was injected to lipodystrophic livers (lanes 3 and 4), but there was little increase in the IRS-2-associated PI3-kinase activity.

The observed reduction of IRS-2 in the livers of lipodystrophic and *ob/ob* mice is a consequence of chronic hyperinsulinemia (Shimomura et al. 2000). This fact was demonstrated in the following studies. Our laboratory measured the mRNA changes in the livers of fasted or refed mice and in streptozotocin-treated, insulin-deficient rats without or with insulin injection. The levels of IRS-2 mRNA rose when insulin levels were reduced either by fasting or streptozotocin treatment. Conversely, IRS-2 mRNA was downregulated when insulin levels were restored either by refeeding or by insulin administration. In addition, when primary rat hepatocytes were cultured in the presence of insulin, the IRS-2 mRNA and protein amounts were reduced in a dose- and time-dependent manner, with

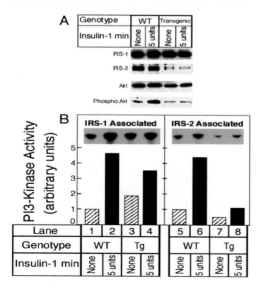

Immunoblot and PI3-Kinase in Livers

Fig. 2. A) Immunoblot analysis of IRS-1, IRS-2, Akt, and Phospho-Akt in livers of wild-type (WT) and transgenic aP2-SREBP-1c lipodystrophic mice. PBS or 5 U of insulin was injected into the portal vein. The liver was excised 1 min after injection and liver lysate was subjected to immunoblot. B) PI3-kinase activities associated with IRS-1 or IRS-2. Liver lysate was immunoprecipitated with antibodies against IRS-1 or IRS-2. Immunoprecipitates were subjected to measurement of PI3-kinase activities. Data from Shimomura et al. (2000) in Panel A. Data in Panel B are unpublished.

no significant alterations in the insulin receptor or IRS-1. Moreover, insulin-mediated stimulation of tyrosine phosphorylation of IRS-2 was diminished, IRS-2-associated PI3-kinase activity decreased, and phosphorylation of Akt was severely diminished (Shimomura et al. 2000). These observations obtained from the primary hepatocyte studies were consistent with the results in livers of lipodystrophic mice with chronic hyperinsulinemia.

A Vicious Cycle

 The experiments described above led to a working model of a vicious cycle that is set up in livers of lipodystrophic and *ob/ob* mice (Fig. 3; Shimomura et al. 2000). According to the model, leptin inhibits insulin secretion, either directly or indirectly (Saufert et al. 1999). In leptin-deficient states, animals oversecrete insulin, due to the leptin deficiency itself, or the overeating that is secondary to leptin deficiency. Once hyperinsulinemia becomes chronic, IRS-2 is downregulated in liver, and this downregulation is associated with a resistance to the normal insulin-mediated repression of gluconeogenesis. Despite the reduction in IRS-2, insulin continues to increase SREBP-1c, which activates the mRNAs for the enzymes that phosphorylate of glucose and its conversion to fatty acids (lipogenesis). The combination of glucose overproduction and enhanced fatty acid synthesis leads to further increases in insulin secretion and resistance, thereby setting up a vicious cycle (Shimomura et al. 2000).

Successful treatment of human generalized lipodystrophy with leptin

Humans with generalized lipodystrophy also have extremely low levels of plasma leptin (Pardini et al. 1998). The studies described above have led to a clinical trial

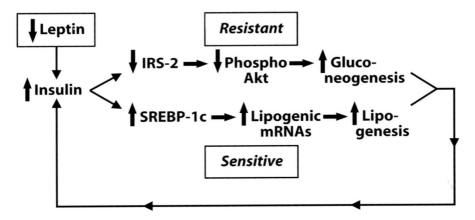

Fig. 3. Model illustrating how hyperinsulinemia secondary to leptin deficiency creates a vicious cycle of insulin resistance and sensitivity coexisting in livers of lipodystrophic and *ob/ob* mice.

designed to determine whether leptin administration to patients with lipodystrophy also reverses the metabolic syndrome of insulin resistance and fatty liver.

Groups at NIH and the University of Texas administered recombinant leptin twice a day for three to four months to nine patients with generalized lipodystrophy who had serum leptin levels of less than 4 ng per milliliter (Oral et al. 2002). The treatment markedly improved hyperglycemia and hypertriglyceridemia. The enlarged liver sizes due to steatosis were reduced by 30 % on average.

The successful treatment of lipodystrophy with leptin encourages leptin-administration to the other types of insulin resistance syndrome, particularly "garden-variety" insulin resistance associated with diet-induced obesity. These common metabolic syndromes, also referred to as syndrome X and abdominal visceral fat-type obesity (DeFronzo 1987; Reaven et al. 1988; Matsuzawa et al. 1995), share the features of leptin resistance and chronic hyperinsulinemia. Therefore, the working model of a vicious cycle in Figure 3 may apply to the more common metabolic syndrome, and the attempt to enhance leptin activity may be a new way to combat insulin resistance syndrome.

References

Brown MS, Goldstein JL (1997) The SREBP pathway: regulation of cholesterol metabolism by proteolysis of a membrane-bound transcription factor. Cell 89:331–340

DeFronzo RA. (1987) Lilly lecture. The triumvirate: beta-cell, muscle, liver. A collusion responsible for NIDDM. Diabetes 37:667–687

Foretz M, Pacot C, Dugail I, Lemarchand P, Guichard C, Le Liepve X, Berthelier-Lubrano C, Spiegelman B, Kim J-T, Ferre P, Foufelle F (1999) ADD1/SREBP-1c is required in the activation of hepatic lipogenic gene expression by glucose. Mol Cell Biol 19:3760–3768

Friedman JM, Halaas JL (1998) Leptin and the regulation of body weight in mammals. Nature 395:763–770

Hall RK, Granner DK (1996) Insulin regulates expression of metabolic genes through divergent signaling pathways. J Basic Clin Physiol Pharmacol 10:119–133

Hillgartner FB, Salati LM, Goodridge AG (1995) Physiological and molecular mechanisms involved in nutritional regulation of fatty acid synthesis. Physiol Rev 75:47–76

Horton JD, Shimomura I (1999) SREBPs: activators of cholesterol and fatty acid biosynthesis. Curr Opin Lipidol 10:143–150

Horton JD, Shimomura I, Brown MS, Hammer RE, Goldstein JL, Shimano H (1998) Activation of cholesterol synthesis in preference to fatty acid synthesis in liver and adipose tissue of transgenic mice overproducing sterol regulatory element-binding protein-2. J Clin Invest 101:2331–2339

Hua X, Yokoyama C, Wu J, Briggs MR, Brown MS, Goldstein JL, Wang X (1993) SREBP-2, a second basic-helix-loop-helix-leucine zipper protein that stimulates transcription by binding to a sterol regulatory element. Proc Natl Acad Sci USA 90:11603–11607

Hua X, Wu J, Goldstein JL, Brown MS, Hobbs HH (1995) Structure of the human gene encoding sterol regulatory element binding protein-1 (SREBF1) and localization of SREBF1 and SREBF2 to chromosomes 17p11.2 and 22q13. Genomics 25:667–673

Kim JB, Spiegelman BM (1996) ADD1/SREBP1 promotes adipocyte differentiation and gene expression linked to fatty acid metabolism. Genes Dev 10:1096–1107.

Kim JB, Sarraf P, Wright M, Kwok MY, Mueller E, Solanes G, Lowell BB, Spiegelman BM (1998) Nutritional and insulin regulation of fatty acid synthetase and leptin gene expression through ADD1/SREBP1. J Clin Invest 101:1–9

Matsuzawa Y, Shimomura I, Nakamura T, Keno Y, Tokunaga K (1995)Pathophysiology and pathogenesis of visceral fat obesity. Ann NY Acad Sci 748: 395–406

O'Brien RM, Granner DK (1996) Regulation of gene expression by insulin. Physiol Rev 76:1109–1161

Oral EA, Simha V, Ruiz E, Andewelt A, Premkumar A, Snell P, Wagner AJ, DePaoli AM, Reitman ML, Taylor SI, Gorden P, Garg A (2002) Leptin-replacement therapy for lipodystrophy. New Engl J Med 346:570–578

Pardini VC, Victoria IM, Rocha SM, Andrade DG, Rocha AM, Pieroni FB, Milagres G, Purisch S, Velho G (1998) Leptin levels, beta-cell function, and insulin sensitivity in families with congenital and acquired generalized lipoatropic diabetes. J Clin Endocrinol Metab 83:503–508

Reaven GM, Hollenbeck C, Jeng CY, Wu MS, Chen YD (1988) Measurement of plasma glucose, free fatty acid, lactate, and insulin for 24 h in patients with NIDDM. Diabetes 37:1020–1024

Saufert J, Klieffer T, Habener JF. (1999) Leptin inhibits insulin gene transcription and reverses hyperinsuinemia in leptin-deficient *ob/ob* mice. Proc Natl Acad Sci USA 96:674–679

Seip M, Trygstad O (1996) Generalized lipodystrophy, congenital and acquired lipoatrophy. Acta Paediatr Suppl 413:2–28

Shimano H, Horton JD, Hammer RE, Shimomura I, Brown MS, Goldstein JL (1996) Overproduction of cholesterol and fatty acids causes massive liver enlargement in transgenic mice expressing truncated SREBP-1a. J Clin Invest 98:1575–1584

Shimano H, Horton JD, Shimomura I, Hammer RE, Brown MS, Goldstein JL (1997) Isoform 1c of sterol regulatory element binding protein is less active than isoform 1a in livers of transgenic mice and in cultured cells. J Clin Invest 99:846–854

Shimomura I, Bashmakov Y, Shimano H, Horton JD, Goldstein JL, Brown MS (1997a) Cholesterol feeding reduces nuclear forms of sterol regulatory element binding proteins in the hamster liver. Proc Natl Acad Sci USA 94:12354–12359

Shimomura I, Shimano H, Horton JD, Goldstein JL, Brown MS (1997b) Differential expression of exons 1a and 1c in mRNAs for sterol regulatory element binding protein-1 in human and mouse organs and cultured cells. J Clin Invest 99:838–845

Shimomura I, Hammer RE, Richardson JA, Ikemoto S, Bashmakov Y, Goldstein JL, Brown MS (1998) Insulin resistance and diabetes mellitus in transgenic mice expressing nuclear SREBP-1c in adipose tissue: model for congenital generalized lipodystrophy. Genes Dev 12:3182–3194

Shimomura I, Bashmakov Y, Horton JD (1999a) Increased levels of nuclear SREBP-1c associated with fatty livers in two mouse models of diabetes mellitus. J Biol Chem 274:30028–30032

Shimomura I, Bashmakov Y, Ikemoto S, Horton JD, Brown MS, Goldstein JL (1999b) Insulin selectively increases SREBP-1c mRNA in livers of rats with streptozotocin-induced diabetes. Proc Natl Acad Sci 96:13656–13661

Shimomura I, Hammer RE, Ikemoto S, Brown MS, Goldstein JL (1999c) Leptin reverses insulin resistance and diabetes mellitus in mice with congenital lipodystrophy. Nature 401:73–76

Shimomura I, Matsuda M, Hammer RE, Bashmakov Y, Brown MS, Goldstein J L (2000) Increased IRS-2 and decreased SREBP-1c leads to mixed insulin resistance and sensitivity in livers of lipodystrophic and ob/ob mice. Mol Cell 6: 77–86

Tontonoz P, Kim JB, Graves RA, Spiegelman BM (1993) ADD1: a novel helix-loop-helix transcription factor associated with adipocyte determination and differentiation. Mol Cell Biol 13:4753–4759

Virkamaki A, Ueki K, Kahn CR (1999) Protein-protein interaction in insulin signaling and the molecular mechanisms of insulin resistance. J Clin Invest 103:931–943

Waters KM, Ntambi JM (1994) Insulin and dietary fructose induce stearoyl-CoA desaturase 1 gene expression of diabetic mice. J Biol Chem 269:27773–27777

Yokoyama C, Wang X, Briggs MR, Admon A, Wu J, Hua X, Goldstein JL, Brown MS (1993) SREBP-1, a basic-helix-loop-helix-leucine zipper protein that controls transcription of the low density lipoprotein receptor gene. Cell 75:187–197

Leptin, Growth and Reproduction

M. L. Aubert, B. Sudre, P. D. Raposinho, D. Vauthay, D. D. Pierroz, and F. P. Pralong[1]

Summary

The elucidation of the *ob/ob* gene product, *leptin*, not only closed a gap in the understanding of the regulation of feeding but also offered a rationale for the humoral link between metabolic function and the regulation of hypothalamo-pituitary secretions. Absence of leptin production as seen in *ob/ob* mice or in some rare cases of human obesity not only leads to hyperphagia, reduced energy expenditure, and hypercorticism, but also, most importantly, to sterility. Partial or total leptin resistance by mutation of the leptin receptor leads to a similar phenotype, as seen in *db/db* mice, *fa/fa* Zucker rats and again in rare cases of human obesity. Common human obesity is characterized by partial resistance to clearly elevated circulating leptin levels. A key finding was the demonstration that treatment of sterile *ob/ob* mice with leptin could quickly restore fertility, implying that a minimum level of circulating leptin is necessary for positive stimulation of the gonadotropic axis, at least as a permissive factor. A similar situation was seen with the treatment of two patients with leptin deficiency. Furthermore, leptin was shown to modulate other hypothalamo-pituitary axes. A general finding has been that leptin administration to animals undergoing severe reduction in energetic supply could reverse the negative effects of such a metabolic insult on most endocrine axes, with striking effects on pulsatile growth hormone (GH) and LH secretions in the rat. Ingestive behavior is controlled by multiple interacting neuroendocrine circuits that are leptin-dependent, involving neuropeptides such as Neuropeptide Y (NPY), Melanocortins (MCs), AGRP, CART, GLP-1, Orexin, etc. Generally speaking, a deficit in feeding corresponds to centrally induced reduction in sexual function. NPY is primarily known to stimulate feeding but also to modulate sexual behavior and gonadotropin secretion. Apparently reproductive function is not dependent on hypothalamic α-MSH or CART action. The recently described natural ligand of the GHRP receptor, ghrelin, which is synthesized and release by the stomach, not only stimulates GH secretion, as predicted, but also regulates feeding by acting on hypothalamic neuropeptides such as NPY. Ghrelin action seems to represent a counterbalance of leptin action. Whereas leptin decreases feeding and can produce anorexia, ghrelin stimulates feeding and eventu-

Division of Biology of Growth and Development, Department of Pediatrics, School of Medicine, 1211 Geneva 14; and Division of Endocrinology and Metabolism[1], Department of Medicine, University School of Medicine, 1011 Lausanne, Switzerland

Kordon et al.
Brain Somatic Cross-Talk and the
Central Control of Metabolism
© Springer-Verlag Berlin Heidelberg 2002

ally produces obesity. Thus a trend for coordinated neuroendocrine regulation of ingestive and reproductive behavior in response to metabolic and environmental changes is expected, with a clear integrative role for leptin and possibly insulin. Still, much remains to be learned about the mode of action of leptin to activate GnRH secretion and reproduction in mammals.

Introduction

The concept that reproductive and anabolic functions depend highly upon nutrition or metabolic conditions related to food intake is logical and well demonstrated, both in human medicine and animal models (Bronson 1986; Foster et al. 1995; Wade et al. 1996; Foster and Nagatani 1999). Timing of puberty has been related to nutrition (Bronson 1986; Frisch 1980). In female subjects, it has been well demonstrated that adequate calorie intake is necessary for allowing normal reproductive cycles to proceed. This requirement was found to be less stringent in males (Bronson 1986). Clearly longitudinal growth and body fat acquisition require normal feeding, with an adequate intake in both calories and proteins. It has been postulated that time of onset of puberty in girls could be best correlated by the acquisition of a minimum amount of fat stores (Frisch 1980), but the mechanisms for transmission of such an effect of body fat on the hypothalamic centers that are responsible for triggering the pubertal release of GnRH pulses have been elusive (Foster and Nagatani 1999). Furthermore, adverse metabolic conditions, such as malnutrition, type-1 diabetes, obesity, lactation, or intensive exercise known to drain most of the energy resources, are associated with reduced or abolished reproductive function secondary to reduction of the hypothalamic drive on gonadotropin secretion (Bronson 1986; Distiller et al. 1975; Steger 1990; Li et al. 1999).

Until recently, the nature of the central mechanisms of inhibition of gonadotropin secretion imposed by such unfavorable metabolic conditions was unclear. The neuroendocrine control of feeding and energy expenditure depends upon a large panel of neuropeptides or neurotransmitters (Schwartz et al. 2000). Among these, POMC gene products such as α-MSH (Thornton et al. 1997), Neuropeptide Y (NPY; Kalra 1993; Pierroz et al. 1996), and Orexin A (Sakurai et al. 1998) are most important. Interestingly, several of the neuropeptides involved in the control of feeding have been found to be implicated in the on and off regulation of reproduction or growth, thus implying a logical relationship between the central regulation of nutrient intake (feeding) and the physiological processes that require additional energy substrates such as growth and reproduction. The discovery, in 1996, of leptin, the hormone encoded by the obesity (*ob*) gene that is a 146 aa protein with a tertiary structure similar to that of cytokines (Zhang et al. 1994), and of ghrelin, in 1999, synthesized in the stomach (Kojima et al. 1999), has provided two links between the periphery and the hypothalamic control of feeding. Clearly, the discovery of leptin has brought a lot of new interesting concepts about the relationship between acquisition of fat stores, metabolic status, and various neuroendocrine functions, in particular those related to the regulation of reproduction and growth. It now appears that leptin represents *a* permissive factor for allowing the reproductive function to occur with a mainly hypothalamic central action. Now the key issue is to understand how leptin affects the neurocircuitry that conditions pulsatile GnRH release, either by a direct action on GnRH neurons or indirectly by the intervention of neuropeptides that are implicated in the regulation of feeding. This last aspect will be mainly addressed in this review. The impact of the recent discovery of ghrelin on our understanding of the control of feeding and possibly some of the neuroendocrine axes is very interesting, but the amount of work with ghrelin is still modest compared to the state of knowledge that has been acquired with leptin studies. Of course, the same questions evoked in the case of leptin exist for ghrelin. This new hormone represents the natural ligand for the growth hormone related protein (GHRP) receptor and thus should primarily affect the regulation of GHRH release and GH secretion but has concomitantly been shown to affect the control of feeding. Our present knowledge about ghrelin will be briefly discussed in the second part of this review.

Leptin and reproduction

The identification of leptin, the product of the gene that is defective in the obese *ob/ob* mouse, has generated an extraordinary interest in the relationship between metabolic status, reproductive function, and the neuroendocrine role of NPY (Zhang et al. 1994; Steiner 1996). The mutation of the leptin gene (*ob*) is responsible for both obesity and sterility in this animal, since treatment with leptin obtained by recombinant technology rapidly reduced food intake and body weight (Zhang 1994) and restored fertility in both sexes (Chehab et al. 1996; Mounzih et al. 1997). There are only a few rare cases of leptin deficiency in the human species. Farooqi et al. (1999) described two patients with a mutation of the leptin gene who reproduced several aspects of the phenotype of the *ob/ob* mouse. Indeed, these children displayed a voracious eating behavior and became grossly obese very early in life. Treatment with recombinant leptin allowed them to immediately normalize this eating disorder and, subsequently, to progressively reduce their body weight. Under leptin treatment, the older patient (9-year-old girl) developed a prepubertal nocturnal, pulsatile release of LH and FSH, whereas the other child (2-year-old boy) corrected his eating behavior upon leptin treatment but did not display any signs of precocious puberty (Farooqi et al. 1999; Farooqi 2002). In one of cases,, leptin was shown to be a permissive factor for the development of puberty in the 9-year-old girl, who shouldnormally start her pubertal development. In the younger patient, leptin administration did not produce precocious puberty, which is a quite important and reassuring observation. Of course the possibility of the absence of pubertal development if no leptin treatment had been given could not be evaluated in this situation. One should recall that two cases of patients with a leptin receptor gene defect have been reported and these patients were found to be completely immature sexually (Strobel et al. 1998; Clement et al. 1998).

Although leptin was thought originally to be exclusively expressed in white adipose tissue, later reports indicated that leptin is expressed in several areas such as the hypothalamus (Morash et al. 1999), pituitary (Jin et al. 2000), fundic gastric epithelium (Bado et al. 1998), skeeletal muscle (Wang et al. 1998), syncy-tiotrophoblast (Masuzaki et al. 1997), and mammary epithelium (Smith-Kirwin et al. 1998). Leptin, mainly of adipocyte origin, is secreted into the general circu-lation and modulates food intake by an action at a central level (Stephens et al. 1995). The concept quickly emerged that leptin controls food intake and repro-duction, at least in part through an action on NPY release (Stephens et al. 1995; Schwartz et al. 1995; Mercer et al. 1996; Rohner-Jeanrenaud et al. 1996), It became evident that other neuropeptides, in addition to NPY, are involved in this process. Indeed, gene expression for most of the other neuropeptides involved in the reg-ulation of feeding was shown to be regulated by leptin, with the orexigenic pep-tides such as NPY, AGRP, and Orexin-A being down-regulated by leptin and the anorectic neuropeptides such as α-MSH, CART or GLP-1 being logically up-regu-lated by leptin. Thus, with the knowledge that leptin activates reproduction, in-volvement of any of these neuropeptides in the regulation of reproduction is pos-sible but needs to be demonstrated.

Leptin has been shown to affect pulsatile secretion of LH in rats, since the dis-appearance of LH pulsatility during fasting can be restored by leptin administra-tion (Nagatani et al. 1998) or indirectly by increasing metabolic fuel oxidation (Schneider et al. 1998). It is expected that leptin secretion would be low or sup-pressed in type-1 IDDM diabetes, since *ob* gene expression in rat adipose tissue is decreased in this situation (Becker et al. 1995). Indeed, leptin secretion is low in streptozotocin-induced type-1 diabetes (Havel et al. 1998; Pierroz et al. 1997), and reciprocally, gene expression for NPY is elevated (Pierroz et al. 1997; Sahu et al. 1992).

Extensive data support the notion that the reproductive actions of leptin are exerted within the hypothalamus. The long form of the leptin receptor that is re-sponsible for signal transduction is heavily expressed in the arcuate nucleus and ventromedial hypothalamus (Elmquist et al. 1998), areas important for control-ling GnRH release and sexual behavior, respectively. Leptin stimulated GnRH re-lease from isolated hypothalamic explants in vitro (Yu et al. 1997; Lebrethon et al. 2000a), and intracerebroventricular (icv) administration of leptin antibodies re-duced pulsatile LH release (Carro et al. 1997a). Also, icv administration of leptin at doses that did not influence peripheral leptin concentrations restored LH se-cretion during fasting in rats (Gruaz et al. 1998a). Taken together, these data sug-gest that leptin acts centrally to influence reproduction but do not answer the question of whether these actions are exerted directly upon GnRH neurons or in-directly through inter-neural inputs.

In addition to these actions of leptin at the hypothalamic level, putative roles of leptin at the pituitary (Zamorano et al. 1997a; Yu et al. 1997; Jin et al. 1999; Iqbal et al. 2000) or gonadal levels (Moschos et al. 2002) have been described, but the physiological meaning of the available observations is still difficult to conceptual-ize. Leptin has been shown to increase LH and FSH release from isolated pitu-itaries in vitro (Yu et al. 1997). Functional leptin receptors have been found in pi-tuitary glands at different ages and conditions (Shimon et al. 1998; Dieterich and Lehnert 1998). Direct inhibitory effects of leptin on cultured granulosa cells from rat and bovine have been described (Zachow and Maggofin 1997; Spicer and Francisco 1998), and full-length leptin receptors have been described in the human ovary (Karlsson et al. 1997). Functional roles for leptin in follicle physiology (Zamorano et al. 1997b; Cioffi et al. 1997) and testicular function (Caprio et al. 1999; Tena-Sempere et al. 1999) have been suggested. Whether direct effects of leptin at these targets are seen normally in vivo, and what these effects would be, are unknown at present. It can nevertheless be postulated that regulation of ovarian (testicular) function by circulating leptin could arise not from minute-to-minute changes in plasma levels but from the permanent changes in concentration range related to alterations in metabolic conditions, with, for example, a modification of gonadal function resulting from continuously low circulating leptin.

Leptin and the control of sexual maturation

It has been hypothesized for a long time that onset of puberty in adolescents would correlate with the acquisition of body mass, fat mass, or other metabolically related factors, which would tell the brain that the body is sufficiently developed to afford the pubertal changes related to the onset of reproductive life (Frisch 1980). This hypothesis implied that a humoral factor would trigger the pubertal increase in gonadotropin secretion; thus the existence of leptin had already been anticipated in 1980. It is known that sexual maturation is delayed when metabolic conditions are not satisfactory, as in food or protein restriction (Kiess et al. 1998; Gruaz et al. 1993). We have shown that central NPY infusion permanently delays sexual maturation (Pierroz et al. 1995), and we suggested that NPY could, at least in part, be responsible for this delay in sexual maturation (Gruaz et al. 1993). The possibility that leptin also controls sexual maturation/function by the same axis has been raised (Cheung et al. 1996; Ahima et al. 1997). Evidence has been provided that NPY could also act as a hypothalamic brake, restraining the onset of puberty in primates (El Majdoubi et al. 2000).

 Delaying sexual maturation: It has been known for a long time that food restriction delays the onset of sexual functions, with females being more sensitive than males. We evaluated the effects of several levels of food restriction on leptin secretion in female rats. Plasma leptin was investigated by radioimmunoassay starting at 24 days of life (d) in normal female rats, and in rats subjected to food restriction. Plasma leptin levels were low at 24 d (289±65 pg/ml) compared to adult levels at 59 d (957±73 pg/ml). Plasma leptin then steadily increased during the juvenile period and reached 740±56 pg/ml at 41 d, at the time of vaginal opening (VO). At this age (41 d), food-restricted rats had no VO and low plasma leptin (19–360 pg/ml). In rats eating 60 % of normal food allowance, spontaneous VO was observed between 55 and 60 d, representing a delay of approximately 20 days, and plasma leptin was 740±48 at 59 d. With a daily food intake reduced to 7–8 g/d (representing 36 % of normal food intake), VO and any kind of reproductive activity were permanently prevented, and plasma leptin concentration was very low. Following a switch to ad libitum feeding at 53 d, plasma leptin immediately increased and reached normal levels after two days. VO occurred four days later (Kiess et al. 1998; Gruaz et al. 1998b). Thus, circulating leptin could represent a signal to the hypothalamus, indicating that nutritional input is compatible with onset of sexual function. To better demonstrate that leptin could represent a permissive factor for the timing of sexual maturation, food-restricted rats received an infusion of mouse leptin (10 μg/d, Lilly) into the lateral ventricle starting at 53 days of life. Such infusion resulted in a small decrease in body weight as compared to food-restricted rats not receiving leptin (91±1 to 80±1 g), suggesting increased energy expenditure. Vaginal opening occurred in eight of nine rats receiving leptin, despite the situation of extreme malnutrition (Gruaz et al. 1998b). Thus leptin clearly can act on the GnRH neuronal system to bring about a "metabolic signal," in this case an inappropriate signal, that puberty can take place.

Advancing sexual maturation: Two groups have demonstrated independently that leptin administration could advance sexual maturation in mice (Cheung et al. 1996; Ahima et al. 1997), and there has been a tendency to extrapolate this finding to other mammalian species. In the normally fed rat, leptin administration did not advance sexual maturation but did partially prevent the negative effects of food restriction induced by leptin on the timing of sexual maturation (Cheung et al. 1996). Infused either centrally or subcutaneously, leptin administration induced a marked, dose-dependent reduction in food intake, resulting in an important reduction of body weight gain. Sexual maturation of pair-fed rats, subjected to a food restriction that matched the restriction induced by leptin, was clearly delayed. Leptin treatment only partially rescued sexual maturation (Gruaz et al. 1998b; Pierroz et al. 1999a), confirming the Cheung et al. (1996) study. There is therefore a clear difference between the mouse and the rat for this effect of leptin on sexual maturation. In a monkey study, Plant and Durrant (1997) could not demonstrate any correlation between the normally elevated plasma leptin levels and onset of pubertal increases in LH and testosterone during puberty in the male monkey. Clearly, a normally elevated secretion of leptin is necessary for onset of pubertal secretion of gonadotropin, but a sudden rise in leptin secretion does not represent the signal for such an increase. The same phenomenon is true for human puberty. The work of Mantzoros et al. (1997) suggests that leptin secretion peaks shortly before puberty in boys. It is our impression that, again like in the monkey, leptin represents a permissive factor for the onset of human sexual maturation, not a signal (Kiess et al. 1998; Blum et al. 1997). Very recently, transgenic mice that overexpress leptin have been developed; they have increased glucose metabolism and insulin sensitivity with, as a result, a complete disappearance of white and brown adipose tissue, thus developing a phenotype of "skinny" mice (Ogawa et al. 1999). Interestingly, these mice have accelerated puberty, perfectly in line with the concept that leptin is promoting early pubertal development in mice (Yura et al. 2000). The counterpart of this observation is that an early onset of hypothalamic hypogonadism was present in these skinny mice, which is highly compatible with the extreme metabolic situation of these female rats and reminiscent of some aspects of the syndrome of hypogonadism in hyperactive women (Yura et al. 2000).

In conclusion, plasma leptin concentration is low after weaning in the female rat and progressively increases during the prepubertal and pubertal periods. In different forms of delayed sexual maturation induced by food restriction, plasma leptin levels remains very low. This is the case for anorexia nervosa patients with amenorrhea (Blum et al. 1997). It is likely that the rising plasma levels of leptin in the prepubertal period represent a permissive factor, indicating that the young animal is metabolically ready to go through the process of sexual maturation. Therefore, our data suggest, at least in the rodent, that leptin could be identified as the long-sought metabolic signal responsible for triggering the onset of puberty **in function of metabolic status.**

Possible targets for the leptin action on reproduction

Whereas it is clear that leptin positively influences the reproductive axis, the challenge remains to understand how it acts, presumably on the GnRH neuronal system, in order to activate this axis. It is not clear whether it acts directly on GnRH neurons or through an indirect action involving the mediation of brain neuropeptides (Foster and Nagatani 1999; Cunningham et al. 1999). The simplest possibility would be that the fat-derived hormone regulates GnRH neuronal activity directly. No real evidence exists of the presence of functional leptin receptors (Ob-Rb) on GnRH neurons. It has been shown that the immortalized GnRH-secreting cell line GT1-7 expresses the long form of leptin receptor, as seen by RT-PCR analysis of total RNA extract from these cells (Magni et al. 1999). Studies on the presence of a leptin receptor gene in the brain of mouse, rat, and monkey by double in situ hybridization have revealed that hypothalamic neurons expressing POMC and NPY coexpress the leptin receptor, whereas no evidence has been obtained that GnRH neurons express this receptor (Cunningham et al. 1999). A direct action of leptin on GnRH neurons is questionable, since it is difficult conceptually to understand how the pattern of change in leptin secretion could alter the feeding behavior and the pulsatile LH release simultaneously. Thus it appears more likely that the action of leptin in the brain is "modulated" through integrative pathways involving several neuropeptides that can then finally act on both feeding centers and GnRH neurons.

a) Leptin, Neuropeptide Y and reproduction

The indication that leptin could regulate reproductive function, possibly by an action mediated by NPY, received immediate attention when treatment of obese *ob/ob* mice with leptin was shown not only to correct their excessive food intake and body weight gain but also to rapidly restore fertility (Chehab et al. 1996; Mounzih et al. 1997) through an activation of the GnRH-LH-gonadal axis (Barash et al. 1996). The description of coexpression of leptin receptor and prepronemropeptide Y mRNA in the arcuate nucleus of mouse hypothalamus (Mercer et al. 1996) has suggested that leptin action on the reproductive axis could be mediated at least in part through an action on NPY neurons. Evidence that hypogonadism is associated with decreased leptin secretion and increased hypothalamic NPY activity has been seen in the case of fasting (Ahima et al. 1996) or delayed puberty (Chehab et al. 1996; Cheung et al. 1996; Pierroz et al. 1995) in rodent models. Of course no data are available in humans.

Hypothalamic NPY, which is tighty regulated by leptin, has been shown to be implicated in the regulation of gonadotropin secretion in several species (Kalra 1993). NPY is synthesized in the arcuate nucleus of the hypothalamus and many other locations in the CNS and appears to control metabolic functions such as food intake and thermogenesis, and also reproductive parameters such as go-nadotropin secretion or sexual behavior (for review, see Kalra 1993 and Pierroz et al. 1996). Intracerebroventricular (icv) injection of NPY has been shown to stim-ulate LH secretion in steroid-intact rats and also to inhibit such secretion in cas-trated rats (Kalra 1993). Five receptor subtypes for NPY have been identified for the transduction of the NPY action (Gehlert 1998). NPY gene expression is in-creased in diabetic rats (Pierroz et al. 1997; Sahu et al. 1992; Williams et al. 1998), and in many other metabolically adverse situations (for review, see Gruaz et al. 1993). We have shown that central infusion of NPY into the lateral ventricle of normal, intact rats rapidly inhibits the gonadotropic axis, leading to an arrest of estrous cyclicity in female rats (Catzeflis et al. 1993) and to major decreases in weight of the seminal vesicle, testis and prostate in male rats in the face of very low testosterone secretion (Pierroz et al. 1996). We have further demonstrated that central NPY infusion completely inhibits the pulsatile secretion of LH, stress-ing the fact that NPY acts centrally to produce hypogonadism (Pierroz et al. 1999b). Chronic NPY infusion also inhibits the gonadotropic axis in mice (Rapos-inho et al. 2001). We have postulated that impaired reproductive function in ad-verse metabolic conditions such as fasting or diabetes could be due to excessive hypothalamic NPY release (Gruaz et al. 1993). In a pharmacological study, we demonstrated that the NPY receptor subtype Y5 apparently is mainly involved in the transduction of the inhibitory NPY action in the rat (Raposinho et al. 1999). Conversely, evidence for a stimulating pathway involving the Y4 receptor has been provided (Jain et al. 1999; Raposinho et al. 2000a). The relationship between leptin action and hypothalamo-pituitary secretions was highlighted by Ahima et al. (1996), who demonstrated that leptin administration prevents the fasting-in-duced neuroendocrine changes. They showed that leptin administration main-tained a normal LH, TSH and ACTH secretion despite fasting by concomitantly preventing the rise in hypothalamic gene expression for NPY that is commonly seen during fasting. The demonstration of this leptin-NPY axis may not be exclu-sively a rodent story, since very recently Plant and colleagues offered a demon-stration that NPY may act as well as a hypothalamic brake, restraining the onset of puberty in their model of male Rhesus monkeys (El Majdoubi et al. 2000).

Two very recent studies with transgenic mice have indicated that the involve-ment of NPY as a tonic inhibitor of sexual function before puberty is rather com-plex. We have shown by a pharmacological approach that the Y5 receptor subtype could be the preferential receptor for the inhibitory effect of NPY on the GnRH-LH axis (Raposinho et al. 1999). Two lines of transgenic mice have been devel-oped lacking either the Y1 (Pedrazzini et al. 1998) or the Y5 receptor gene (Marsh et al. 1998). These two lines of transgenic mice exhibit normal fertility, implying that with one Y receptor missing, no real consequence on reproduction occurs. Age of VO was identical between transgenic and wild-type mice (Pralong et al. 2002). With the knowledge that leptin administration can advance sexual matura-tion in the mouse, early administration of leptin to Y1-lacking mice was able to advance VO to a much larger extent compared to wild-type controls, whereas no such effect was seen with the transgenic mice lacking the Y5 receptor (Pralong et al. 2002). The removal of the Y1 receptor thus represents a facilitatory effect for leptin action. In this circumstance, the Y1 receptor seems to be the receptor mediating the temporary inhibition of onset of pulsatile GnRH release before puberty in the mouse. In this mouse, puberty occurs prematurely only if the Y1 is absent **and** leptin levels are grossly elevated.

An embarassing story about the putative NPY receptor that modulates the inhibitory action of NPY on reproduction came from a study performed by crossbreeding transgenic mice lacking the Y4 receptor and *ob/ob* mice that are sterile because of lack of leptin. For these double knockout mice ($Y4^{-/-}$,ob/ob; in other words, no leptin and no functional Y4 receptor), the obesity phenotype was not affected, but lack of the Y4 receptor in this *ob/ob* background (no leptin) curiously rescued fertility in male *ob/ob* mice and in half of the female *ob/ob* mice (Sainsbury et al. 2002). Thus the Y4 receptor, known to be a "stimulatory" receptor for the action of NPY on reproduction in the rat (Jain et al. 1999; Raposinho et al. 2000a)), appears now to be an inhibitory receptor. One should recall nevertheless that studies with transgenic mice should be analyzed only with caution, since reorganization of the assignment of different receptor subtypes that are pleiotropic may lead to a "normal" function and therefore provide a false interpretation of the role of each of these receptors in normal mice.

b) Leptin, the melanocortin system and reproduction

Among other regulators of ingestive behavior that are regulated by leptin, melanocortin (MC) peptides such as α-MSH are known to induce satiety, presumably through the MC4 receptor subtype, and jointly or independently, to alter energy expenditure through an action on MC3 and/or MC3 receptors (Cone 1999). Disruption of the MC4 receptor system, either by null mutation (Huszar et al. 1997) or by constant antagonism of this receptor subtype (Cone 1999; Fan et al. 1997; Ollmann et al. 1997; Small et al. 2001), results in hyperphagia, maturity-onset obesity, hyperinsulinemia and hyperglycemia (Cone 1999). Aberrations in pigmentation have also been described. The question remains whether activation of the MC4 receptor subtype in the situation of elevated leptin secretion may be required to activate the reproductive axis and thus transduce a leptin message into modifications of GnRH release. The genetic models of disruption of this receptor subtype have always yielded animals that are fertile, thus indicating that this receptor is not essential for leptin action. Furthermore, morbid obesity associated with melanocortin 4 receptor deficiency in human patients has been associated with hyperphagia, a tendency toward tall stature, and hyperinsulinemia, but preserved reproductive function (Farooqi et al. 2000).

Using a seven-day infusion into the lateral ventricle of male rats with either the MC3/4 receptor antagonist SHU9119 or porcine NPY (10 nmol/d), we were able to produce in both cases an important obesity syndrome. As expected, icv infusion of NPY produced a profound hypogonadism, whereas the obesity syndrome induced by permanent blockade of the MC4 receptor subtype was not associated with any form of decreased reproductive function (Raposinho et al. 2000b). Thus, in the first analysis, the melanocortin signaling system that is regulated by leptin does not appear to control reproduction. This concept is consistent with data published by Hohmann et al. (2000), who addressed the same question by using the otherwise sterile *ob/ob* mouse that becomes fertile upon leptin treatment (Chehab et al. 1996; Mounzih et al. 1997). They co-administered the MC antagonist SHU9119 with leptin to *ob/ob* mice and obtained the same process of initiation of sexual function as when leptin is administered alone. In contrast, leptin's effects on feeding and body weight gain were attenuated in the presence of the MC4 receptor antagonist (Hohmann et al. 2000). Taken together these observations make it unlikely that α-MSH and the melanocortin system play a significant role in the transduction of leptin action on the gonadotropic axis.

c) Leptin, CART and reproduction

CART (cocaine- and amphetamine-regulated transcript), a brain-located peptide, represents another satiety factor stimulated by leptin action, as is the case for POMC derivatives. Food-deprived animals show a pronounced decrease in expression of CART mRNA in the arcuate nucleus. In animal models of obesity with disrupted leptin signalling such as *ob/ob* mice, CART mRNA is almost absent from the arcuate nucleus and peripheral administration of leptin stimulates CART mRNA expression. An antiserum against CART increases feeding in normal rats, indicating that CART may be an endogenous inhibitor of food intake. When injected icv into rats, recombinant CART peptide inhibits both normal and starvation-induced feeding and completely blocks the feeding response induced by NPY (Kristensen et al. 1998). To further assess CART's role as an anorectic signal, CART-deficient mice were generated by gene targeting (Asnicar et al. 2001). On a high fat diet, CART-deficient and female heterozygote mice showed significantly increased food consumption, body weight gain and fat accumulation. Thus CART deficiency predisposed mice to become obese but clearly to a much lower extent than with any genetic disruption along the melanocortin system, thus ranking CART as a less important anorectic factor than α-MSH. As for the other neuropeptides involved in the control of feeding, the same question is whether CART is involved, one way or another, in the regulation of the gonadotropic axis. Using cultured rat hypothalamus, Lebrethon et al. (2000b) showed that CART was able to mediate the stimulatory effect of leptin on the rat GnRH pulse generator, a model in which specific actions of leptin and NPY on GnRH release had been demonstrated (Lebrethon et al. 2000a). They showed that an anti-CART serum prevents the stimulatory action of leptin on the GnRH pulse generator and that CART is able to reduce the GnRH interpulse interval, which represents an activation in this system. They further showed in their in vitro system that the hypothalamic GnRH pulse generator of Zucker (*fa/fa*) rats that are insensitive to leptin can be directly activated by CART (Lebrethon et al. 2000b). These data suggest that CART could be one down-stream mediator of the leptin stimulatory action on the gonadotropic axis. Unfortunately no in vivo demonstration has yet been provided for such a positive action. In this respect, it appears that the CART-deficient mice described by Asnicar et al. (2001), despite becoming obese, were fertile and were able to raise normal- sized litters. Thus removal of an anorectic peptide such as α-MSH or CART produces the same effect of obesity without affecting reproductive competence.

d) Leptin, orexin and the neuroendocrine control of reproduction

Orexin A and B (ORX; Sakurai et al. 1998) or hypocretins (De Lecea et al. 1998) are recently discovered novel neuropeptides that have been implicated in feeding (Sakurai et al. 1998; Sakurai 1999) and drinking behaviors (Kunii et al. 1999), as well as neuroendocrine functions (Date et al. 1999; van den Pol et al. 1998). ORX receptor mRNA has been localized in the ventromedial hypothalamic nucleus (VMH), paravenricular nucleus (PVN), tena tecta, hypocampal formation, dorsal raphe and locus coeruleus in the rat (Trivedi et al. 1998). These areas are involved in food intake and neuroendocrine functions. Central injections of ORX enhance food intake (Sakurai et al. 1998; Sakurai 1999), suppress prolactin release (Russell et al. 2000), and may suppress (Tamura et al. 1999) or stimulate (Pu et al. 1998) LH secretion in the rat. Fasting upregulates ORX mRNA expression (Sakurai et al. 1998), and leptin treatment inhibits this response (Lopez et al. 2000). The long form of the leptin receptor (Ob-Rb) is found in ORX cells (Hakansson et al. 1999) and leptin treatment regulates ORX mRNA levels (Lopez et al. 2000). Thus ORX represents another orexigenic, leptin-regulated neuropeptide that displays mixed functions, acting on feeding and the reproductive axis. Recently Russell et al. (2001) further demonstrated in the rat important interactions for Orexin A with the hypothalamo-pituitary axis pertaining to reproduction. In particular, ORX A stimulated GnRH release in hypothalamic explants harvested from male rats or female rats at proestrous. Female hypothalami harvested at other stages of the ovarian cycles were insensitive to ORX action. An interaction between ORX and NPY action was found since a specific NPY Y1 antagonist abolished in vitro release of GnRH by ORX A, implying that NPY interacts with ORX for this action. Recently, Iqbal et al. (2001) presented evidence that ORX-containing neurons provide direct input to GnRH neurons in the ovine hypothalamus. Dual labeling demonstrated widespread expression of the long form of the leptin receptor within all ORX cells. A third of the GnRH neurons that were examined had ORX immunoreactive terminals in close contact. Thus this study in sheep suggests an integral role for ORX in the regulation of GnRH neurons in the sheep and possibly provides evidence for a novel mechanism whereby leptin and ORX can influence reproductive neuroendocrine function. The possibility exists that ORX neurons could integrate several signals, including the leptin signal, to provide specific inputs to the GnRH neurons.

Leptin and the neuroendocrine control of growth

Although not immediately recognized, leptin appears to control the neuroendocrine circuit that modulates GH secretion (Carro et al. 1997; Vuagnat et al.

1998); thus it could in one way or another influence longitudinal growth. GH secretion is basically regulated by the differential release of GHRH and somatostatin (Guillemin et al. 1982). Although the first studies with leptin did not immediately indicate that leptin could also modulate the neuroendocrine control of GH secretion by an action on GHRH neurons (Ahima et al. 1996), it became evident that, at least in the rodent, normally elevated plasma levels for leptin represent a permissive factor for GH secretion, as is the case for gonadotropin secretion (Carro et al. 1997b; Vuagnat et al. 1998). Low or absent leptin secretion represents a situation of inadequate nutrition or altered energetic homeostasis, like in type 1 diabetes. In this situation, there is no need for a physiologically relevant GH secretion to promote growth and anabolic processes that could lead to unnecessary drain of energetic substrates. Thus leptin could signal the brain that adequate GH secretion can take place and anabolic processes are possible because of adequate energy supply. Central administration of leptin antiserum led to a decrease in GH secretion in the rat. Leptin administration by a central route did not modify GH secretion in normally fed rats, but prevented the disappearance of GH secretion related to fasting (Carro et al. 1997b). In a similar approach, central infusion of leptin to rats submitted to starvation for three days fully prevented the loss of pulsatile GH release (Vuagnat et al. 1998). In this study, the loss of GH secretion during fasting was clearly correlated with collapse of endogenous leptin secretion. Furthermore, whereas fasting was associated with an increase in hypothalamic gene expression for NPY, a fact that could be predicted, the central leptin administration prevented this NPY increase, thus suggesting that elevated NPY release represents an inhibitory signal to GHRH neurons. We subsequently showed that constant NPY central infusion to male rats fully inhibits the somatotropic axis with, as primary event, the full inhibition of hypothalamic GHRH gene expression (Raposinho et al. 2000b). Thus, as for GnRH neurons, leptin appears to act indirectly on GHRH neurons. Central administration of leptin to hypophysectomized fasting rats increased GHRH mRNA levels and decreased somatostatin mRNA content, confirming a role for GHRH and somatostatin as mediators for leptin-induced secretion (Carro et al. 1999). Evidence that leptin can act specifically on somatostatin release to monitor GH secretion was provided by an in vitro study in which leptin given in physiological amount could inhibit low glucose-induced somatostatin secretion in perfused adult hypothalami (Quintela et al. 1997). These data indicated that leptin can rescue GH secretion in malnourished rodents but do not tell whether extra leptin could enhance GH secretion and growth. Tannenbaum et al. (1998) showed that by infusing murine leptin into normally fed rats, leptin enhanced spontaneous pulsatile GH secretion and the GH response to GHRH. There are few data on leptin action on GH secretion in higher species, for example in humans, but it can be predicted that leptin represents a permissive factor for proper stimulation of the somatotropic axis and growth in man.

Ghrelin, a new peripheral hormone opposing the effects of leptin

The ghrelin story is very interesting for two reasons: first because it provided an interesting end to the search for a growth hormone related peptide (GHRP) or GH secretagogue (GHS), independent of GHRH, and second because it provided a peripheral hormonal factor that acts in an inverse fashion to leptin on the hypothalamic regulation of food intake. In the early 1980s, several small peptides were found to release GH by an action in both the hypothalamus and the pituitary.They were called GHRPs (Bowers et al. 1980). They were thought to be analogues of a natural ligand that would provide stimulation of GH release in addition to the action of the hypothalamic GHRH 44 aa peptide found in 1982. An orphan, G-protein coupled receptor was later found to represent the GHRP receptor (Howard et al. 1996). A systematic search for a natural ligand for this receptor culminated with the discovery of a 28-amino acid peptide synthesized and released by the stomach. This peptide was named ghrelin (Kojima et al. 1999). As its name implies, ghrelin is a GH secretagogue, able to stimulate GH release. In line with previous observations that GHRP would stimulate feeding, ghrelin was found to specifically stimulate feeding by an action on NPY. Thus ghrelin stimulates feeding and energy production and signals directly to the hypothalamic regulatory nuclei that control energy homeostasis (Inui 2001). In particular, ghrelin appears to stimulate NPY synthesis and release by antagonizing leptin action at the hypothalamic level (Shintani et al. 2001; Horvarth et al. 2001). Icv ghrelin injection causes a dose-related increase in food intake in rats. This effect is abolished when a NPY Y1 antagonist is co-injected. The leptin-induced inhibition of food-intake can be reversed in a dose-dependent manner by ghrelin (Shintani et al. 2001). In contrast, ghrelin administration has no effect on POMC gene expression, although this last point deserves further study. Ghrelin may have an interesting role in body weight regulation. Data on circulating ghrelin in obese patients are still controversial (Tschop et al. 2001).

Although a great deal of work is still necessary to integrate the differential role of ghrelin and leptin, there are interesting facts that should be mentioned. These two hormones are secreted in a pulsatile fashion, with fasting augmenting all parameters of ghrelin pulsatile secretion and diminishing leptin secretion by selectively attenuating the pulse amplitude; concomitantly, fasting produced synchrony in ghrelin and leptin pulse discharge (Bagnasco et al. 2002). Whereas leptin administration is known to produce anorexia, chronic ghrelin administration caused hyperphagia and obesity in rats. Such an effect was obtained only if ghrelin was injected in the arcuate or paraventricular nucleus (Wren et al. 2001). These effects of chronic administration of ghrelin to the rat are reminiscent of those obtained by chronic, central infusion of NPY, which also produces obesity (Pierroz et al. 1997). Thus, it appears that continued administration of ghrelin permanently drives NPY release and produces the unabated increase in food intake with, as a consequence, a rapid increase in body weight gain and fat deposition.

More work is clearly needed to integrate the specific contributions of leptin and ghrelin and the interaction of these peripheral peptides, to understand the neuroendocrine regulation of feeding and growthn and to delineate the dysregulations of this dual control that could explain pathophysiological situations.

Conclusions

Inappropriate metabolic conditions result in hypothalamic hypogonadism, both in rodent models and in higher species, including humans. Invariably, the adverse metabolic conditions lead to suppression of the GnRH drive on gonadotrophin secretion. Only the threshold for such a suppressive effect varies from species to species, or according to age or gender. The same concept is true for the regulation of growth in function of the metabolic situation, since inadequate nutritional conditions lead to suppression of GHRH pulsatile release, the hypothalamic drive of GH secretion. Less clear are the mechanisms of suppression of pulsatile release of GnRH or GHRH. Obviously, these mechanisms include several factors, and probably there are redundant pathways that make their analysis difficult.

Whereas now two peripheral hormones have been identified, leptin and ghrelin, that clearly modulate feeding, energy expenditure, and neuroendocrine pathways at the hypothalamic level, the roles of glucose (Bucholtz et al. 1996) and insulin in such a capacity should not be forgotten. Insulin secretion and tissue sensitivity to insulin action are two key features of balanced energetic metabolism, and "adverse metabolic conditions" are most often linked with either suppressed insulin secretion, like in type 1 diabetes, or inappropriately increased basal insulin secretion, like in obesity and in the early phase of type 2 diabetes with, as a consequence, development of insulin insensitivity. In this context, insulin and leptin are hypothesized to be "joint adiposity signals" for the long-term regulation of body weight by the brain (Baskin et al. 1999). Accordingly, changes in plasma levels of leptin or insulin mirror a state of normal or altered energy homeostasis and adiposity, and the brain responds by adjusting food intake to restore adipose tissue mass to a regulated level. Before the identification of leptin, insulin was postulated to penetrate the brain and to act on the expression of the neuropeptides involved in the regulation of feeding, such as NPY (Schwartz et al. 1992). Now insulin appears to affect feeding principally by modulating leptin secretion. Nevertheless, the concept that insulin could represent a significant regulator of both feeding and neuroendocrine function was reinforced with the description of the phenotype of transgenic mice that carry a neuron-specific disruption of the insulin receptor gene (NIRKO mice; Brüning et al. 2000). Inactivation of the insulin receptor had no impact on brain development or neuronal survival, but produced expected metabolic alterations such as diet-sensitive obesity, mild insulin resistance, and elevated insulin levels. Most strikingly, NIRKO mice exhibited a clear phenoytpe of hypogonadism with impaired spermatogenesis and ovarian follicle maturation because of hypothalamic dysfunction of LH secretion. Thus insulin might also bring an integrative signal to the brain to enable reproductive function to proceed, or alternatively, GnRH neurons may need an insulin support in order to be operational.In this case, any form of insulin insensitivity is deleterious to the expression of normal hypothalamic activity of the GnRH neurons. More attention should be paid to insulin action within the hypothalamus and its role in the maintenance of neuroendocrine secretions.

In summary, the prevailing concepts about the metabolic control of reproduction and growth have been clearly revolutionized by the discoveries of: leptin and ghrelin and their roles in metabolic parameters such as food intake; the role of NPY and other neuropeptides as possible neurotransmitters of the hypothalamic action of leptin and ghrelin; the role of insulin in this context; and, finally, the striking observations that leptin tone represents a permissive factor for maintenance of reproductive function or GH secretion.

Acknowledgments

The authors wish to acknowledge the excellent technical assistance of Anne Scherrer, Audrey Aebi, Sandrine Jaccard-Duffey, Jean-Pierre Giliberto, and Brigitte Delavy. We are very much in debt to our secretary Céline Gonseth, who helped us in many aspects of the work performed in our research unit. The skillful technical assistance of Jean-Jacques Goy and Ramon Junco in our animal quarter is gratefully acknowledged. This study was supported by a grant from the Swiss National Research Science Foundation 31-55732.98, and 31-67'194.01, and partly by Ferring Research.

References

Ahima RS, Prabakaran D, Mantzoros C, Qu D, Lowell B, Maratos-Flier E, Flier JS (1996) Role of leptin in the neuroendocrine response to fasting. Nature 382:250–252

Ahima RS, Dushay J, Flier SN, Prabakaram D, Flier JS (1997) Leptin accelerates the onset of puberty in normal female mice. J Clin Invest 99:391–395

Asnicar MA, Smith DP, Yang DD, Heiman ML, Fox N, Chen YF, Hsiung HM, Köster A (2001) Absence of Cocaine- and Amphetamine-Regulated Transcript in obesity in mice fed a high calorie diet. Endocrinology 142:4394–4400

Bado A, Levasseur S, Attoub S, Kermorgant S, Laigneau J-P, Bortoluzzi M-N, Moizo L, Lehy T, Guerre-Millo, Le Marchand-Brustel Y, Lewin MJM (1998) The stomach is a source of leptin. Nature 394: 790–794

Bagnasco M, Kalra PA, Kalra SP (2002) Ghrelin and leptin pulse discharge in fed and fasted rats. Endocrinology 143:726–729

Barash IA, Cheung CC, Weigle DS, Ren H, Kabitting EB, Kuijer JL, Clifton DK, Steiner RA (1996) Leptin is a metabolic signal to the reproductive system. Endocrinology 137:3144–3147

Baskin DG, Lattemann DF, Seeley RJ, Woods SC, Porte D Jr, Schwartz MW (1999) Insulin and leptin: dual adiposity signals to the brain for the regulation of food intake and body weight. Brain Res 848:114–123

Becker DJ, Ongemba LN, Brichard V, Henquin JC, Brichard SM (1995) Diet- and diabetes-induced changes of ob gene expression in rat adipose tissue. FEBS Letters 371:324–328

Blum WF, Englaro P, Hanitsch S, Juul A, Hertel NT, Muller J, Skakkebaek NE, Heiman ML, Birkett M, Attanasio A, Kiess W, Rascher W (1997) Plasma leptin levels in healthy children and adolescents: dependence on body mass index, body fat mass, pubertal stage, and testosterone. J Clin Endocrinol Metab 82:2904–2910

Bowers CY, Momany F, Reynolds GA, Chang D, Hong A, Chang K (1980) Structure-activity relationships of a synthetic pentapeptide that specifically releases growth hormone in vitro. Endocrinology 106:663–667

Bronson FH (1986) Food-restricted, prepubertal female rats: rapid recovery of luteinizing hormone pulsing with excess food and full recovery of pubertal development with gonadotropin-releasing hormone. Endocrinology 118: 2483–2487

Brüning JC, Gautam D, Burks DJ, Gillette J, Schubert M, Orban DJ, Klein R, Krone W, Müller-Wieland D, Kahn CR (2000) Role of brain insulin receptor in control of body weight and reproduction. Science 289:2212–2125.

Bucholtz DC, Vidwans NM, Herbosa CG, Schillo KK, Foster DL (1996) Metabolic interfaces between growth and reproduction V. Pulsatile LH secretion is dependent upon glucose availability. Endocrinology 137:601–607

Caprio M, Isidori AM, Carta AR, Moretti C, Dufau ML, Fabbri A (1999) Expression of functional leptin receptors in rodents Leydig cells. Endocrinology 140:4939–4947

Carro E, Pinilla L, Seoane LM, Considine RV, Aguilar E, Casanueva FF, Dieguez C (1997a) Influence of endogenous leptin tone on the estrous cycle and luteinizing hormone pulsatility in female rats. Neuroendocrinology 66:375–377

Carro E, Senaris R, Considine RV, Casanueva FF, Dieguez C (1997b) Regulation of in vivo growth hormone secretion by leptin. Endocrinology 138:2203–2206

Carro E, Senaris RM, Seoane LM, Frohman LA, Arimura A, Casanueva FF, Dieguez C (1999) Role of growth hormone (GH)-releasing hormone and somatostatin on leptin-induced GH secretion. Neuroendocrinology 69:3–10

Catzeflis C, Pierroz DD, Rohner-Jeanrenaud F, Rivier J, Sizonenko PC, Aubert ML (1993) Neuropeptide Y administered chronically into the lateral ventricle profoundly inhibits both the gonadotropic and the somatotropic axis in intact adult female rats. Endocrinology 132:224–234

Chehab FF, Mounzih K, Lu R, Lim ME (1996) Early onset of reproductive function in normal mice treated with leptin. Science 275:88–90

Chehab F, Lim M, Lu R (1997) Correction of the sterility defect in homozygous obese female mice by treatment with the human recombinant leptin. Nature Genet 12:318–320

Cheung CC, Thornton JE, Kuijper JL, Weigle DS, Clifton DK, Steiner RA (1996) Leptin is a metabolic gate for the onset of puberty in the female rat. Endocrinology 138:855–858

Cioffi JA, Van Blerkom J, Antczak M, Shafer A, Wittmer S, Snodgrass HR (1997) The expression of leptin and its receptors in the pre-ovulatory human follicles. Mol Human Reprod 3:467–472

Clement K, Vausse C, Lahalo N, Cabrol S, Pelloux V, Cassuto D, Gourmelen M, Dina C, Chambaz J, Lacorte JM, Basdevant A, Bougneres P, Lebouc Y, Froguel P & GuyGrand B (1998) A mutation in the human leptin receptor gene causes obesity and pituitary dysfunction. Nature 392:398–401

Cone RD (1999) The central melanocortin system and energy homeostasis. Trends Endocrinol Metab 10:211–216

Cunningham MJ, Clifton DK, Steiner RA (1999) Leptin's action on the reproductive axis: perspectives and mechanisms. Biol Reprod 60:216–222

Date Y, Ueta Y, Yamashita H, Yamaguchi H, Matsukura S, Kangawa K, Sakurai T, Yanagisawa M, Nakazato M (1999) Orexins, orexigenic hypothalamic peptides, interact with autonomic, neuroendocrine and neuroregulatory systems. Proc Natl Acad Sci USA 96:748–753.

de Lecea L, Kilduff TS, Peyron C, Gao X, Foye PE, Danielson PE, Fukuhara C, Battenberg EL, Gautvik VT, Bartlett FS 2nd, Frankel WN, van den Pol AN, Bloom FE, Gautvik KM, Sutcliffe JG (1998) The hypocretins: hypothalamus-specific peptides with neuroexcitatory activity. Proc Natl Acad Sci USA 95:322–327

Dieterich KD, Lehnert H (1998) Expression of leptin receptor mRNA and the long form splice variant in human pituitary and pituitary adenoma. Exp Clin Endocrinol Diabetes 106:522–525

Distiller LA, Sagel J, Morley JE, Joffe BI, Seftel HC (1975) Pituitary responsiveness to luteinizing hormone-releasing hormone in insulin-dependent diabetes mellitus. Diabetes 24:378–380

El Majdoubi M, Sahu A, Ramaswamy, Plant TM (2000) Neuropeptide Y: a hypothalamic brake restraining the onset of puberty in primates. Proc Natl Acad Sci USA 97:6179–6184

Elmquist JK, Bjorbaek C, Ahima RS, Flier JS, Saper CB (1998) Distribution of leptin receptor mRNA isoforms in the rat brain. J Comp Neurol 395:535–547

Fan W, Boston BA, Kesterson RA, Hruby, VJ, Cone RD (1997) Role of melanocortinergic neurons in feeding and the Agouti obesity syndrome. Nature 385:165–168

Farooqi IS (2002) Leptin and the onset of puberty: insights from rodent and human genetics. Semin Reprod Med 20:139–144

Farooqi IS, Jebb SA, Langmack G, Lawrence E, Cheetham CH, Prentice AM, Hughes IA, McCamish MA, O'Rahilly S (1999) Effects of recombinant leptin therapy in a child with congenital leptin deficiency. N Engl J Med 341:879–884

Farooqi IS, Yeo GSH, Keogh JM, Aminian S, Jebb SA, Butler G, Cheetham T, O'Rahilly S (2000) Dominant and recessive inheritance of morbid obesity associated with melanocortin 4 receptor deficiency. J Clin Invest 106: 271–279

Foster DL, Bucholtz DC, Herbosa CG (1995) Metabolic signals and the timing of puberty in sheep. In: Plant TM and Lee PA (eds) The neurobiology of puberty. Bristol, UK, J Endocrinol, pp. 243–257

Foster DL, Nagatani S (1999) Physiological perspectives on leptin as a regulator of reproduction: role in timing puberty. Biol Reprod 60: 205–215

Frisch RE (1980) Pubertal adipose tissue: is it necessary for normal sexual maturation? Fed Proc 39:2395–2400

Gehlert DR (1998) Multiple receptors for the pancreatic polypeptide (PP-fold) family: physiological implications. Proc Soc Exper Biol Med 218:7–22

Gruaz NM, Pierroz DD, Rohner-Jeanrenaud F, Sizonenko PC, Aubert ML (1993) Evidence that neuropeptide Y could represent a neuroendocrine inhibitor of sexual maturation in unfavorable metabolic conditions in the rat. Endocrinology 133:1891–1895

Gruaz NM, Lalaoui M, Pierroz DD, Raposinho PD, Blum WF, Aubert ML (1998a) Failure of leptin administration to advance sexual maturation in the female rat. 80th Annual Meeting of the Endocrine Society. New Orleans, Louisiana, Abstract P3–668

Gruaz NM, Lalaoui M, Pierroz DD, Englaro P, Sizonenko PC, Blum WF, Aubert ML (1998b) Chronic administration of leptin into the lateral ventricle induces sexual maturation in severely food-restricted female rats. J Neuroendocrinol 10:627–633

Guillemin R, Brazeau P, Bohlen P, Esch F, Ling N, Wehrenberg WB (1982) Growth hormone-releasing factor from a human pancreatic caused acromegaly. Science 218:585–587

Hakansson M, de Lecea L, Sutcliffe JG, Yanagisawa M, Meister B (1999) Leptin receptor- and STAT3-immunoreactivities in hypocretin/orexin neurones of the lateral hypothalamus. J Neuroendocrinol 11:653–663

Havel PJ, Uriu-Hare Y, Liu T, Stanhope KL, Stern JS, Keen CL, Ahren B (1998) Marked and rapid decreases of circulating leptin in Streptozotocin diabetic rats: reversal by insulin. Am J Physiol 274: R1482–R1491

Hohmann JG, Teal TH, Clifton DK, Davis J, Hruby VJ, Han G, Steiner RA (2000) Differential role of Melanocortin in mediating leptin's central effects on feeding and reproduction. Am J Physiol 278:R50–R59

Horvarth TL, Diano S, Sotonyi P, Heiman M, Tschop M (2001) Minireview: ghrelin and the regulation of energy balance-a hypothalamic perspective. Endocrinology 142:4163–4169

Howard AD, Feighner SD, Cully DF, Arena JP, Liberator PA, Rosenblum CI, Hamelin M, Hreniuk DL, Palyha OC, Anderson J, Paress PS, Diaz C, Chou M, Liu KK, McKee KK, Pong SS, Chaung LY, Elbrecht A, Dashkevicz M, Heavens R, Rigby M, Sirinathsinghji DJ, Dean DC, Melillo DG, Patchett AA, Nargund R, Griffin PR, DeMartino JA, Gupta SK, Schaeffer JM, Smith RG, Van der Ploeg LH, (1996) A receptor in pituitary and hypothalamus that functions in growth hormone release. Science 273:974–977

Huszar D, Lynch CA, Fairchild-Huntress V, Dunmore JH, Fang Q, Berkemeier LR, Gu W, Kesterson RA, Boston BA, Cone RD, Smith FJ, Campfield LA, Burn P, Lee F(1997) Targeted disruption of the melanocortin-4 receptor results in obesity in mice. Cell 88:131–141

Iqbal J, Pompolo S, Considine RV, Clarke IJ (2000) Localization of leptin receptor-like immunoreactivity in the corticotropes, somatotropes, and gonadotropes in the ovine anterior pituitary. Endocrinology 141:1515–1520

Iqbal J, Pompolo S, Sakurai T, Clarke IJ (2001) Evidence that Orexin-containing neurons provide direct input to Gonadotropin-Releasing Hormone neurons in the ovine hypothalamus. J Neuroendocrinol 13:1033–1041

Inui A (2001) Ghrelin: an orexigenic and somatotrophic signal from the stomach. Nature Rev 2:1–10

Jain MR, Pu S, Kalra PS, Kalra SP (1999) Evidence that stimulation of two modalities of pituitary luteinizing hormone release in ovarian steroid-primed rats may involve neuropeptide Y Y1 and Y4 receptors. Endocrinology 140:5171–5177

Jin L, Burguera BG, Couce ME, Scheithauer BW, Lamsan J, Eberhardt NL, Kulig E, Lloyd RV (1999) Leptin and leptin receptor expression in normal and neoplastic human pituitary: evidence of a regulatory role for leptin on pituitary cell proliferation. J Clin Endocrinol Metab 84:2903–2909

Jin L, Zhang S, Burguera BG, Couce ME, Osamura RY, Kulig E, Lloyd RV (2000) Leptin and leptin receptor expression in rat and mouse pituitary cells. Endocrinology 141:333–339

Kalra SP (1993) Mandatory neuropeptide-steroid signaling for the preovulatory luteinizing-hormone-releasing hormone discharge. Endocrinol Rev 14:507–538

Karlsson C, Lindell K, Svenssonh E, Bergh C, Lind P, Billig H, Carlsson LS, Carlsson B (1997) Expression of functional leptin receptors in the human ovary. J Clin Endocrinol Metab 82:4144–4148

Kiess W, Blum WF, Aubert ML (1998) Leptin, puberty and reproductive function: lessons from animal studies and observations in humans. Eur J Endocrinol 138: 26–29

Kojima M, Hosoda H, Date Y, Nakazato M, Matsuo H, Kangawa K (1999) Ghrelin is a growth hormone releasing acylated peptide from stomach. Nature 402:656–660

Kristensen P, Judge ME, Thim L, Ribel U, Christjansen KN, Wulff BS, Clausen JT, Jensen PB, Madsen OD, Vrang N, Larsen PJ, Hastrup S (1998) Hypothalamic CART is a new anorectic peptide regulated by leptin. Nature 393:72–76

Kunii K, Yamanaka A, Nambu T, Matsuzaki I, Goto K, Sakurai T (1999) Orexins/hypocretins regulate drinking behaviour. Brain Res 842:256–261

Lebrethon MC, Vandersmissen E, Gérard A, Parent AS, Junien JL, Bourguignon J-P (2000a) In vitro stimulation of the prepubertal rat gonadotropin-releasing hormone pulse generator by leptin and neuropeptide Y through distinct mechanisms. Endocrinology 141:1464–1469

Lebrethon MC, Gérard A, Parent AS, Bourguignon JP (2000b) Cocaine and amphetamine-regulated transcript peptide mediation of leptin stimulatory effect on the rat gonadotropin-releasing hormone pulse generator in vitro. J of Neuroendocrinology 12:383–386

Li C, Chen P, Smith MS (1999) Identification of neuronal input to the arcuate nucleus (ARH) activated during lactation: implications in the activation of neuropeptide Y neurons. Brain Res 824:267–276

Lopez M, Seoane L, Garcia MC, Lago F, Casanueva FF, Senaris R, Dieguez C (2000) Leptin regulation of prepro-orexin and orexin receptor mRNA levels in the hypothalamus. Biochem Biophys Res Commun 269:41–45

Magni P, Vettor R, Pagano C, Calcagno A, Beretta E, Mesdsi E, Zanisi M, Martini L, Motta M (1999) Expression of a leptin receptor in immortalized gonadotropin-releasing hormone-secreting neurons. Endocrinology 140:1581–1585

Mantzoros CS, Flier JS, Rogol AD (1997) A longitudinal assessment of hormonal and physical alterations during normal puberty in boys. V. Rising leptin levels may signal the onset of puberty. J Clin Endocrinol Metab 82:1066–1070

Marsh DJ, Hollopeter G, Kafer KE, Palmiter RD (1998) Role of the Y5 neuropeptide Y receptor in feeding and obesity. Nature Med 4:718–721

Masuzaki H, Ogawa Y, Sagawa N, Hosofda K, Matsumoto T, Mise H, Nishimura H, Yoshimasa Y, Tanaka I, Mori T, Nakao K (1997) Nonadipose tissue production of leptin: leptin as a novel placenta-derived hormone in humans. Nature Med 3:1029–1033

Mercer JG, Hoggrad N, Williams LM, Lawrence CB, Hannah LT, Morgan PJ, Trayhurn P (1996) Coexpression of leptin receptor and preproneuropeptide Y mRNA in arcuate nucleus of mouse hypothalamus. J of Neuroendocrinology 8:733–735

Morash B, Li A, Murphy PR, Wilkinson M, Ur E (1999) Leptin gene expression in the brain and pituitary gland. Endocrinology 140:5995–5998

Moschos S, Chan JL, Mantzoros CS (2002) Leptin and reproduction: a review. Fertility and Sterility 77:433–444

Mounzih K, Lu R, Chehab FF (1997) Leptin treatment rescues the sterility of genetically obese ob/ob males. Endocrinology 138:1190–1193

Nagatani S, Guthikonda P, Thompson RC, Tsukamura H, Maeda K-I, Foster DL (1998) Evidence for GnRH regulation by leptin: Leptin administration prevents reduced pulsatile LH secretion during fasting. Neuroendocrinology 67:370–376

Ogawa Y, Masuzaki H, Hosoda K, Aizawa-Abe M, Suga J, Suga M, Ebihara K, Iwai H, Matsuoka N, Satoh N, Odaka H, Kasuga H, Fujisawa Y, Inoue G, Nishimura H, Yoshimasa Y, Nakao K. (1999) Increased glucose metabolism and insulin sensitivity in transgenic skinny mice over-expressing leptin. Diabetes 48:1822–1829

Ollmann MM, Wilson BD, Yang YK, Kerns JA, Chen Y, Gantz I, Barsh GS (1997) Antagonism of central melanocortin receptors in vitro and in vivo by agouti-related protein. Science 278:135–138

Pedrazzini T, Seydoux J, Kunstner P, Aubert JF, Grouzmann E, Beermann F, Brunner HR (1998) Cardiovascular response, feeding behavior and locomotor activity in mice lacking the NPY Y1 receptor. Nature Med 4:722–726

Pierroz DD, Gruaz NM, d'Allèves V, Aubert ML (1995) Chronic administration of neuropeptide Y into the lateral ventricle starting at 30 days of life delays sexual maturation in the female rat. Neuroendocrinology 61:293–300

Pierroz DD, Catzeflis C, Aebi AC, Rivier JE, Aubert ML (1996) Chronic administration of neuropeptide Y into the lateral ventricle inhibits both the pituitary-testicular axis and growth hormone and insulin-like growth factor-I secretion in intact adult male rats. Endocrinology 137:3–12

Pierroz DD, Héritier A, Lalaoui M, d'Allèves V, Blum WF, Aubert ML (1997) Leptin is a metabolic signal for sexual function: reciprocal changes in plasma leptin and arcuate nucleus NPY mRNA in two models of adverse metabolic conditions with hypogonadism. The Endocrine Society, 79th Annual Meeting, June 1997, Abstract OR24-6

Pierroz DD, Gruaz-Gumowski NM, Lalaoui M, Blum WF, Aubert ML (2000) Leptin and NPY regulation of sexual maturation in the rat. In: Bourguignon JP and Plant TM (eds), the Onset of Puberty in Perspective. Elsevier, Amsterdam, pp 339–349

Pierroz DD, Aebi A, Huhtaniemi IT, Aubert ML (1999b) Many LH peaks are needed to physiologically stimulate testosterone secretion: modulation by fasting and NPY. Am J Physiol 276:E603–E610

Plant TM, Durrant AR (1997) Circulating leptin does not appear to provide a signal for triggering the initiation of puberty in the male rhesus monkey (Macaca Mulatta). Endocrinology 138:4505–4508

Pralong FP, Gonzales C, Voirol MJ, Palmiter RD, Brunner HR, Gaillard RC, Seydoux J, Pedrazzini T (2002) The neuropeptide Y Y1 receptor regulates leptin-mediated control of energy homeostasis and reproductive functions. FASEB J. 16:712–714

Pu S, Jain MR, Kalra PS, Kalra SP (1998) Orexins, a novel family of hypothalamic neuropeptides, modulate pituitary luteinizing hormone secretion in an ovarian steroid-dependent manner. Regul Pept 78:133–136

Quintela M, Senaris R, Heiman ML, Casanueva FF, Dieguez C (1997) Leptin inhibits in vitro hypothalamic somatostatin secretion and somatostatin mRNA levels. Endocrinology 138:5641–5644

Raposinho PD, Broqua P, Pierroz DD, Hayward A, Dumont Y, Quirion R, Junien JL, Aubert ML (1999) Evidence that the inhibition of LH secretion exerted by central administration of

Neuropeptide Y (NPY) in the rat is predominantly mediated by the NPY-Y5 receptor subtype. Endocrinology 140:4046–4055

Raposinho PD, Broqua P, Hayward A, Akinsanya K, Galyean R, Schteingart C, Junien JL, Aubert ML (2000a) Stimulation of the gonadotropic axis by the neuropeptide Y receptor Y1 antagonist/Y4 agonist 1229U91 in the male rat. Neuroendocrinology 71:2–7

Raposinho PD, Castillo E, d'Allèves V, Broqua P, Pralong FP, Aubert ML (2000b) Chronic blockade of the Melanocortin 4 receptor subtype leads to obesity independently of Neuropeptide Y action, with no adverse effects on the gonadotropic and somatotropic axes. Endocrinology 141:4419–4427

Raposinho PD, Pierroz DD, Broqua P, White RW, Pedrazzini T, Aubert ML (2001) Chronic administration of neuropeptide Y into the lateral ventricle of C57BL/6J male mice produces an obesity syndrome including hyperphagia, hyperleptinemia, insulin resistance, and hypogonadism. Mol Cellular Endocrinol 185:195–204

Rohner-Jeanrenaud F, Cusin I, Sainsbury A, Zakrzewska KE, Jeanrenaud B (1996) The loop system between Neuropeptide Y and leptin in normal and obese rodents. Horm Metab Res 28:642–648

Russell SH, Kim MS, Small CJ, Abbott CR, Morgan DG, Taheri S, Murphy KG, Todd JF, Ghatei MA, Bloom SR (2000) Central administration of orexin A suppresses basal and domperidone stimulated plasma prolactin. J Neuroendocrinol 12:1213–1218

Russell SH, Small CJ, Kennedy AR, Stanley SA, Seth A, Murphy KG, Taheri S, Ghatei MA, Bloom SR (2001) Orexin A interactions in the hypothalamo-pituitary gonadal axis. Endocrinology 142: 5294–5302

Sahu A, Sninsky CA, Phelps CP, Dube MG, Kalra PS, Kalra SP (1992) Neuropeptide-Y release from the paraventricular nucleus increases in association with hyperphagia in streptozotocin-induced diabetic rats. Endocrinology 131:2979–2985

Sainsbury A, Schwartzer C, Couzens M, Jenkins A, Aokes SR, Ormandy CJ, Herzog H (2002) Y4 receptor knockout rescues fertility in ob/ob mice. Genes Dev 16:1077–1088

Sakurai T (1999) Orexins and orexin receptors: implication in feeding behavior. Regul Pept 85:25–30

Sakurai T, Amemiya A, Ishii M, Matsuzaki I, Chemelli RM, Tanaka H, Williams SC, Richardson JA, Kozlowski GP, Wilson S, Arch JR, Buckingham RE, Haynes AC, Carr SA, Annan RS,McNulty DE, Liu WS, Terrett JA, Elshourbagy NA, Bergsma DJ, Yanagisawa M (1998) Orexins and orexin receptors: a family of hypothalamic neuropeptides and G protein-coupled receptors that regulate feeding behavior. Cell 92:573–585

Schneider JE, Goodman MD, Tang S, Bean B, Ji H, Friedman MI (1998) Leptin indirectly affects estrous cycles by increasing metabolic fuel oxidation. Horm Behav 33:217–228

Schwartz MW, Figlewicz, Baskin DG, Woods SC, Porte D Jr (1992) Insulin in the brain: A hormonal regulator of energy balance. Endocrinol Rev 13:387–414

Schwartz MW, Baskin DG, Bukowski TR, Kuijper JL, Foster D, Lasser G, Prunkard DE, Porte Jr D, Woods SC, Seeley RJ, Weigle DS (1995) Specificity of leptin action on elevated blood glucose levels and hypothalamic neuropeptide Y gene expression in ob/ob mice. Diabetes 45:531–535

Schwartz MW, Woods SC, Porte D Jr, Seeley RJ, Baskin DG (2000) Central nervous system control of food intake. Nature 404:661–671

Shimon I, Yan X, Magoffin DA, Friedman TC, Melmed S (1998) Intact leptin receptor is selectively expressed in human fetal pituitary and pituitary adenomas and signals human fetal pituitary growth hormone secretion. J Clin Endocrinol Metab. 83:4059–4064

Shintani M, Ogawa Y, Ebihara K, Aizawa-Abe M, Miyanaga F, Takaya K, Hayashi T, Inoue G, Hosoda K, Kojima M, Kangawa K, Nakao K (2001) Ghrelin, an endogenous growth hormone secretagogue, is a novel orexigenic peptide that antagonizes leptin action through the activation of hypothalamic neuropeptide Y/Y1 receptor pathway. Diabetes 50:227–232

Small CJ, Kim MS, Stanley SA, Mitchell JRD, Murphy K, Morgan DGA, Ghatei MA, Bloom SR (2001) Effects of chronic central nervous system administration of Agouti-related protein in pair-fed animals. Diabetes 50:248–254

Smith-Kirwin SM, O'Connor DM, De Johnston J, Lancey ED (1998) Leptin expression in human mammary epithelial cells and breast milk. J Clin Endocrinol Metab 83:1810–1813

Spicer LJ, Francisco CC (1998) Adipose obese gene product, leptin, inhibits bovine ovarian thecal cell steroidogenesis. Biol Reprod 58:207–212

Steger RW (1990) Neuroendocrine and reproductive consequences of diabetes mellitus in the male. In: Shafrir E (ed) Frontiers in diabetes research. Lessons from animal diabetes III. Smith-Gordon, pp. 529–537

Steiner RA (1996) Editorial: Lords and Ladies Leapin' on leptin. Endocrinology 137:4533–4534

Stephens TW, Basinski M, Bristow PK, Bue-Valleskey JM, Burgett SG, Craft L, Hale J, Hofmann J, Hsiung HM, Kriauciunas A, MacKellar W, Rosteck PR, Schoner B, Smith D, Tinsley FC, Zhang XY, Heiman M (1995) The role of Neuropeptide Y in the antiobesity action of the obese gene product. Nature 377:530–532

Strobel A, Issad T, Camoin L, Ozata M, Strosberg AD (1998) A leptin missense mutation associated with hypogonadism and morbid obesity. Nature Genet 18: 213–215

Tamura T, Irahara M, Tezuka M, Kiyokawa M, Aono T (1999) Orexins, orexigenic hypothalamic neuropeptides, suppress the pulsatile secretion of luteinizing hormone in ovariectomized female rats. Biochem Biophys Res Commun 264:759–762

Tannenbaum GS, Gurd W, Lapointe M (1998) Leptin is a potent stimulator of spontaneous pulsatile growth hormone (GH) secretion and the GH response to GH-releasing hormone. Endocrinology 139:3871–3875

Tena-Sempere M, Pinilla L, Gonzalez LC, Dieguez C, Casanueva FF, Aguilar E (1999) Leptin inhibits testosterone secretion from adult rat testis in vitro. J Endocrinol 161:211–218

Thornton JE, Cheung CC, Clifton DK, Steiner RA (1997) Regulation of hypothalamic proopiomelanocortin mRNA by leptin in ob/ob mice. Endocrinology 138: 5063–5066

Trivedi P, Yu H, MacNeil DJ, Van der Ploeg LH, Guan XM (1998) Distribution of orexin receptor mRNA in the rat brain. FEBS Lett 438:71–75

Tschop M, Meyer C, Tataranni PA, Devanarayan V, Ravussin E, Heiman ML (2001) Circulating ghrelin levels are decreased in human obesity. Diabetes 50:707–709

van den Pol AN, Gao XB, Obrietan K, Kilduff TS, Belousov AB (1998) Presynaptic and postsynaptic actions and modulation of neuroendocrine neurons by a new hypothalamic peptide, hypocretin/orexin. J Neurosci 18:7962–7971

Vuagnat BAM, Pierroz DD, Lalaoui M, Pralong FP, Blum WF, Aubert ML (1998) Evidence for a Leptin-Neuropeptide Y axis for the regulation of Growth Hormone secretion in the rat. Neuroendocrinology 67:291–300

Wade GN, Schneider JE, Li H-Y (1996) Control of fertility by metabolic cues. Am J Physiol 270:E1–E19

Wang J, Liu R, Hawkins M, Barzilai N, Rossetti L (1998) A nutrient-sensing pathway regulates leptin gene expression in muscle and fat. Nature 394:790–793

Williams G, Steel JH, Cardoso H, Ghatei MA, Lee YC, Gill JS, Burrin JM, Polak JM, Bloom SR (1998) Increased hypothalamic neuropeptide Y concentrations in diabetic rats. Diabetes 37:763–772

Wren AM, Small CJ, Abbott CR, Dhillo WS, Seal LJ, Cohen MA, Batterman RL, Taheri S, Stanley SA, Ghatei MA, Bloom SR (2001) Ghrelin causes hyperphagia and obesity in rats. Diabetes 50:2540–2547

Yu WH, Kimura M, Walczewska A, Karanth S, McCann SM (1997) Role of leptin in hypothalamic-pituitary function. Proc Natl Acad Sci USA 94:1023–1028

Yura S, Ogawa Y, Sagawa N, Nasuzaki H, Itoh H, Ebihara K, Aizawa-Abe M, Fujii S, Nakao K (2000) Accelerated puberty and late onset hypothalamic hypogonadism in female transgenic skinny mice overexpressing leptin. J Clin Invest 105:749–755

Zachow RJ, Maggofin DA (1997) Direct intraovarian effect of leptin: impairment of the synergistic action of insulin-like growth factor-I on follicle stimulating hormone-dependent estradiol-17β production by rat ovarian granulosa cells. Endocrinology 138: 847–850

Zamorano PL, Mahesh VB, De Sevilla LM, Chorich LP, Bhat GK, Brann DW (1997a) Expression and localization of the leptin receptor in endocrine and neuroendocrine tissues of the rat. Neuroendocrinology 65: 223–228

Zamorano PL, Zachow RJ, Magoffin DA (1997b) Direct intraovarian effects of leptin: impairment of the synergistic action of the insulin-like growth factor I on follicle-stimulating hormone-dependent estradiol-17 beta production by rat ovarian granulosa cells. Endocrinology 138:847–850

Zhang Y, Proenca R, Maffei M, Barone M, Loepole L, Friedman J (1994) Positional cloning of the mouse obese gene and its human homologue. Nature 372:425–432

An Emerging Role of Leptin in Clinical Psychiatry

T. Pollmächer[1]

Summary

Early in the 20th century changes in appetite and weight had already been recognized as important features of severe psychiatric disorders. The present chapter reviews recent evidence suggesting that the fat cell-derived hormone leptin is pathophysiologically involved in these changes. Moreover, data are discussed supporting the speculation that leptin, which is now recognized to be a cytokine-like peptide involved in many aspects of brain function such as neurodevelopment, neuronal survival and various aspects of behavior and cognition, plays a pathophysiological role in behavioral and cognitive changes observed in psychiatric patients and, in particular, in anorexia nervosa and schizophrenia.

Introduction

Changes in food intake and weight during the course of severe psychiatric disorders were already recognized at the turn of the 20th century. Emil Kraepelin, in particular, emphasized that psychotic disorders such as manic-depressive illness (bipolar affective disorder) or dementia praecox (schizophrenia) are eventually accompanied by substantial weight loss. Moreover, across the relapsing-remitting course of these disorders weight may show dramatic fluctuations. In an early case description (Kraepelin 1901), Kraepelin presented a depressive patient who, in the first 1.5 years of the disorder, lost more than 35 kg of weight and later on showed fluctuations within individual episodes of up to 25 kg. In addition, Kraepelin noted that fluctuations in weight did not occur at random but that weight loss was related to a deterioration in the psychiatric condition and weight gain to an improvement in the psychiatric condition. Furthermore, he noted that, in general, weight gain was not a mere consequence of the patient's improved condition but clearly preceded clinical improvement. This early empirical discovery suggests that networks regulating appetite, food intake and metabolism, and finally weight might be linked to the pathophysiology of severe psychiatric disorders.

In the present chapter we will discuss this link from one particular perspective, which is the potential role of the adipose tissue hormone leptin in the pathophysiology of psychiatric disorders. We chose to address leptin (Auwerx and

---

[1]Max Planck Institute of Psychiatry, Krapelinstrasse 10, D-80804 Munich, Germany

Kordon et al.
Brain Somatic Cross-Talk and the
Central Control of Metabolism
© Springer-Verlag Berlin Heidelberg 2002

Staels 1998) because this cytokine-like substance, in addition to its pivotal role in signaling the size of the adipose tissue to the brain and inducing adaptive changes in food intake, has been shown to be involved in a set of other behaviors that are often disturbed in psychiatric patients, e.g., sexuality, sleep and motor activity, suggesting a quite widespread involvement in brain function. Therefore, leptin seems to be a very interesting candidate peptide for a presumed link between the regulation of weight and psychiatric disorders.

After briefly recapitulating the physiology of leptin we will take three examples (anorexia nervosa, schizophrenia, and changes in weight induced by antipsychotic drugs) to illustrate the idea that alterations in the circulating amounts of leptin in psychiatric patients do not just reflect changes in weight but might in addition be important for the understanding of other abnormalities in brain function in these patients. Due to the very few data available in this field, the ideas presented here are quite speculative and are meant to stimulate further research rather than to overinterpret available evidence.

Leptin – regulation of food intake and beyond

Leptin was discovered in 1994 and has attracted incredible scientific attention ever since. By now more than 5000 scientific publications have appeared addressing the structure, production and function of this 167-amino acid protein. Leptin is the product of the *ob* gene which was cloned and shown to be defective in an obese mouse strain (Zhang et al. 1994). Leptin is produced mainly by adipose tissue, although there is evidence that the production might also occur within the brain (Esler et al. 1998). The actions of leptin are mediated through splice variants of a specific receptor that is a class I cytokine receptor (Auwerx and Staels 1998). This class of receptors also includes those for interleukin-2 (IL-2), interferons and growth hormone. Downstream signals include janus kinase 2 and STAT 3,5 and 6.

One important function of leptin, which actually led to its name, derived from the Greek word λερτοσ meaning "thin", is to signal the size of adipose tissue to the brain. The levels of leptin in peripheral blood are closely and positively correlated to the body mass index (BMI, calculated as weight divided by the square of the height in meters) and to fat mass (Kalra et al. 1999). Obesity in animals with a defective leptin gene or a defective leptin receptor suggests that leptin reduces food intake and fat mass. Indeed, obesity induced by leptin deficiency in rodents and humans can be successfully corrected by leptin administration (Farooqi et al. 1999). However, in people with obesity unrelated to defects in the leptin system, leptin has only slight weight-reducing effects, probably due to a relative leptin resistance (Heymsfield et al. 1999).

The main target for the actions of leptin in the brain is the hypothalamus, where leptin receptors are densely expressed. Here, the leptin signal meets almost every known neuropeptide and neurotransmitter system, and all of them are directly or indirectly involved in the regulation of food consumption, energy expenditure and metabolism (see Fig. 1). Due to the dense interactions of all kinds of neuromodulators, it is not surprising that leptin affects additional brain func-

Hypothalamus

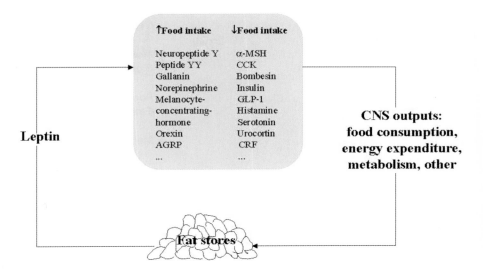

Fig. 1. Leptin as peripheral signal from the adipose tissue to the hypothalamus (adapted from Kraus et al. 2001).

tions (see Fig. 2) regulated by the hypothalamus such as the neuroendocrine systems (Wauters et al. 2000), reproduction (Köpp et al. 1997), motor activity and sleep-wake behavior (Sinton et al. 1999). In addition to these behavioral effects, preliminary evidence suggests that leptin is also involved in cognitive processes (Shanley et al. 2001), has neuroprotective effects (Dicou et al. 2001) and is involved in brain development. Leptin-deficient animals have small brains, an abnormality that can be corrected by leptin administration (Steppan and Swick 1999).These effects of leptin fit well with the idea that leptin is a cytokine. This classification is even more obvious when considering some of its peripheral effects on hematopoiesis and the immune system (Fantuzzi and Faggioni 2000) as well as bone formation (Karsenty 2001).

This short sketch of the physiology of leptin suggests that this peptide is not only a pivotal signal in the networks regulating food intake and weight but is also involved in brain development, neuronal survival, cognition and in almost every basic brain function regulated by the hypothalamus. The hypothalamus relays these functions tightly to mood, anxiety, thought, perception and cognition, which are dysfunctional in psychiatric disorders. Hence, it seems reasonable to view the pathophysiological role of leptin in psychiatric disorders from a broader point of view than just the one of weight regulation. Below we will attempt to do this in three different areas where some – although preliminary – data are available.

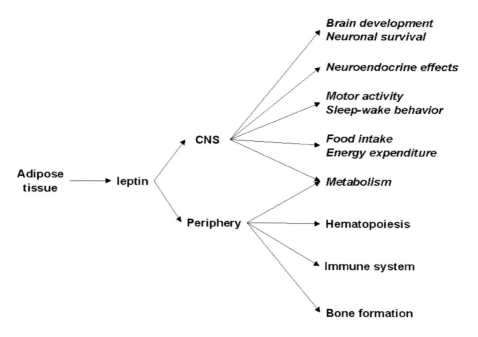

Fig. 2. Functions of leptin (adapted from Auwerx and Staels 1998).

Leptin in anorexia nervosa

Anorexia nervosa (Hebebrand et al. 1999) is the best-recognized eating disorder and occurs in 1 % of the female population in developed countries. Males are sometimes affected but their relative risk is at least 15 times lower compared to females. The peak incidence of the disorder is between 14 and 17 years of age. The overall mortality is high (about 10 %), in part due to extremely low body weight but also to additional psychiatric disorders such as personality disorders or substance abuse or dependence. The major diagnostic symptoms are low body weight and amenorrhea. According to diagnostic criteria the BMI must be below 17.5 kg/m^2 but often drops below 10 kg/m^2. Even at this stage of severe anorexia, patients frequently report feeling overweight, indicating a pronounced distortion of the body image. The disorder is characterized by deliberately induced weight loss, which is achieved by restriction of food intake, intake of laxatives and/or vomiting. Moreover, patients tend to massively increase motor activity (Beumont et al. 1994), which is interpreted as a deliberate attempt to increase energy expenditure.

In accordance with low body weight, leptin levels are drastically reduced in patients with anorexia nervosa, and leptin might be almost undetectable in patients with extremely low BMIs (Köpp et al. 1998). It is astonishing that despite this kind of acquired, nearly total, leptin deficiency, patients are still able to fast. Upon refeeding leptin levels often rise sharply, suggesting some kind of a rebound effect.

Recent evidence suggests that the lack of leptin is a pivotal factor for amenor-rhea (Köpp et al. 1997) and, in addition, reduced availability of leptin might con-tribute to hematological abnormalities (anemia, granulocytopenia, thrombope-nia) in anorexia nervosa (Devuyst et al. 1993). Moreover, the leptin deficiency in these patients might also be involved in changes in motor activity: in obese and normal animals administration of leptin promotes motor activity. This makes sense because increased motor activity supports leptin-induced weight loss. However, increased motor activity makes physiological sense not only in obesity but also in starvation, albeit for a different reason, which is the necessity to search for food. Hence, it is not surprising that, in rats put on a food restriction regime, motor activity is dramatically enhanced. However, it is surprising that in these starved animals leptin almost completely blocks the increase in motor activity (Exner et al. 2000). Hence, a leptin deficiency as it occurs during starvation might be a signal to enhance the output of motor systems. Therefore, leptin might play an important role in the disturbed motor behavior of patients with anorexia ner-vosa. This does not mean that psychological factors such as the reasoning that in-creased activity supports weight loss are not important, but leptin could support a vicious cycle initiated by these factors: initially, the patients would deliberately increase motor behavior to lose weight; then, along with the weight loss, a de-creasing leptin production would render the drive for increased motor activity self-sustaining and more or less independent of active efforts.

Hence, motor activity, which so far has been thought to be exclusively under active control of patients suffering from anorexia nervosa, might be caused or sustained by a physiological consequence of starvation, which is leptin deficiency. It would be worthwhile to test this hypothesis by studying the effects of leptin ad-ministration on motor activity in patients with anorexia nervosa.

Leptin in schizophrenia

Schizophrenia (Bukanan 2000) is a brain disorder that severely deteriorates nu-merous complex functions of the central nervous system, including thought, emotion, perception, cognition and behavior. Due to the high lifetime prevalence of over 1 %, the onset in early adulthood and the tendency towards chronicity, the disorder requires a very high degree of health care provisions. About one quarter of hospital beds are occupied by schizophrenic patients, and the total costs of treatment are enormous (e.g., $ 50 billion per year in the United States). Although there is no cure for schizophrenia, the combined use of pharmacological and psy-chosocial interventions considerably improves outcome, enhances the quality of life of the patients affected, and, to a large extent, makes social integration possi-ble (Pollmächer 2002).

However, it is still a most important challenge for psychiatric research to un-ravel the causes of schizophrenia. Definitively, schizophrenia is of multifactorial origin. There is clear evidence demonstrating a strong genetic component, al-though no particular genes causing schizophrenia have been found so far (Maier et al. 1999). Probably the minor effects of multiple genes are important, rather than large effects of single genes. Environmental factors involved include pre-

and perinatal complications of various origins, including maternal infections. Brain morphology and histology are not grossly abnormal, but there is converging evidence suggesting subtle brain damage compatible with either a disturbance of neurodevelopment and/or a subtle neurodegenerative process starting in childhood or early adulthood (Lieberman 1999).

Epidemiological studies suggest that schizophrenic patients as a group do not show abnormalities in weight (Allison et al. 1999a). However, on an individual basis, it is evident that weight might show huge fluctuations depending on the prevailing symptomatology and medication (see section below). Patients having delusions of being persecuted or poisoned might stop eating for long times and lose considerable weight. Patients with a prominent negative symptomatology, which includes decreased motivation and motor activity and sometimes increased food intake, may be significantly overweight.

So far, only one study has investigated the levels of circulating leptin in schizophrenic patients. We compared leptin levels of 42 subjects suffering from schizophrenia to those of 64 healthy controls (Kraus et al. 2001). After controling for age, gender, BMI, medication and smoking behavior, leptin levels were almost 50 % below the mean value in controls. Leptin levels were also below those of a psychiatric control group that consisted of patients suffering from depression.

It is somewhat surprising to find such a prominent reduction of leptin levels in schizophrenia, and there has been no convincing explanation for this finding so far. Because the patients were acutely ill and were studied on the day following hospital admission, stress effects might play a role. However, glucocorticoids, which are pivotal stress mediators, enhance leptin levels (Newcomer et al. 1998), and Cushing patients with a chronic hyperactivity of the hypothalamo-pituitary-adrenal axis show increased levels as well (Masuzaki et al. 1997). On the other hand, particular stressors might even reduce leptin secretion, mainly via adrenergic pathways (Rayner and Trayhurn 2001) and independently of the HPA system (Schafroth et al. 2001). Hence, the evidence regarding the influence of stress on leptin levels is somewhat equivocal. Moreover, a successful treatment of schizophrenia with classical antipsychotic drugs does not go along with an increase in leptin levels (Kraus et al. 1999) suggesting that the reduced levels we observed are unlikely to be a transient phenomenon related to hospitalization stress.

Speculating on the presumed pathophysiological significance of leptin deficiency in schizophrenia, at present, two explanations appear quite attractive: 1) cognitive deficits are pivotal symptoms of schizophrenia. Very recently, it was shown that leptin can support long-term potentiation, a basic neurophysiological mechanism important for various cognitive functions, by facilitating NMDA receptor transmission (Shanley et al. 2001). Hence, leptin deficiency could contribute to cognitive dysfunctions in patients with schizophrenia; 2) the present concepts about the origin of schizophrenia assume that, due to unknown reasons, neurodevelopmental or neurodegenerative processes occur (Lieberman 1999). Leptin deficiency might be involved in both of these processes since leptin is necessary for proper brain development (Steppan and Swick 1999) and has a neuroprotective effect (Dicou et al. 2001). Future studies should test concrete hypotheses derived from these speculations which might even be driven further by studies suggesting that leptin deficiency in schizophrenia may be corrected by some antipsychotic drugs currently in use. These studies will be described in the following section.

Leptin and antipsychotic drugs

Studies about the effects of antipsychotic drugs, which are mainly used to treat schizophrenic patients, on leptin levels were recently performed to understand a troublesome side effect of a number of these drugs, which is weight gain. This effect has been known since the introduction of the first antipsychotics in the 1950s (Kraus et al. 2001). However, weight gain is particularly prominent with some of the newer, second generation drugs such as clozapine and olanzapine. With these two drugs the mean weight gain over 10 weeks has recently been estimated to be approximately 4 kg (Allison et al. 1999b). Individual patients, though, may gain 20–30 kg over 6–12 months. Some patients develop a strong carbohydrate craving almost immediately after the treatment is started (Brömel et al. 1998). The increase in body weight is probably due to an increase in body fat without changes in lean mass (Eder et al. 2001).

Both olanzapine and clozapine have been shown to induce prominent increases in plasma leptin levels (see Fig. 3), which do not occur in patients who re-

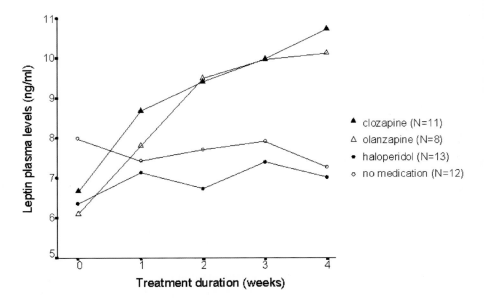

Fig. 3. The influence of various antipsychotic drugs on plasma leptin levels in psychiatric patients. Drugs that induce weight gain (olanzapine and clozapine) induce prominent increases in leptin levels during the first two weeks of treatment. Haloperidol, which does not induce weight gain, has no effect on leptin levels either. These also remain stable in patients who are not pharmacologically treated over four weeks. Data taken from Kraus et al. 1999.

Table 1. Influence of various psychotropic drugs on weight in psychiatric patients. Note that despite weight gain some drugs do not or hardly affect leptin levels.

Drug	Mean effect on weight over 4–6 weeks	Effect on plasma leptin levels
Antipsychotic drugs (Kraus et al. 1999)		
Clozapine	+3.9 kg	Prominent increase during the first 2 weeks
Olanzapine	+3.1 kg	Prominent increase during the first 2 weeks
Haloperidol	No significant change	No significant change
Antidepressant drugs (Hinze-Selch et al. 2000; Kraus et al. 2002)		
Amitriptyline	+3.5 kg	No significant change
Mirtazapine	+2.4 kg	Slight increase after 4 weeks
Paroxetine	No significant change	No significant change

ceive conventional drugs devoid of effects on weight (Kraus et al. 1999). This finding is not surprising due to the well established correlation between fat mass and leptin levels. However, a steeply increased leptin production during treatment with olanzapine and clozapine occurs prior to a significant increase in weight. Moreover, other psychotropic drugs that induce weight gain have no or only slight effects on leptin production (see Table 1). Due to these findings it is very unlikely that increased leptin levels during treatment with second generation antipsychotic drugs are simply a consequence of increased food intake and weight gain.

Antipsychotic drugs are potent blockers of various neurotransmitter receptors (Pickar 1995). Among these, histamine and serotonin receptors are particularly involved in the regulation of appetite and food intake. Because the effects of leptin on feeding require an intact histaminergic system (Morimoto et al. 2001), the dramatic increase in leptin production induced by second generation antipsychotic drugs might reflect a central leptin resistance due to a histamine H1 receptor blockage. However, as shown in Table 1, amitriptyline, which induces weight gain to a similar extent as olanzapine or clozapine, is also a potent H1 blocker but does not increase leptin production. Hence, it is likely that leptin plays a role in drug-induced weight gain but the particular reasons for the effects of second generation antipsychotic drugs on leptin secretion and the details of the role of leptin in drug-induced changes in weight remain to be clarified.

Again, we would like to speculate at this point somewhat beyond weight regulation in a different direction: there is circumstantial evidence that weight gain is a positive predictor of the clinical efficacy of clozapine (Bustillo et al. 1996; Jalenques et al. 1996). This positive effect of weight gain is presumably an indirect one, which could, for example, be related to an increased availability of leptin. This sounds particularly interesting in the context of the reduced leptin levels we found in patients upon hospital admission and the growing evidence that leptin might be involved in neurodevelopment, neuronal survival and cognition. The latter effect is also interesting in view of the fact that the second generation drugs, and in particular clozapine, seem to be more potent in patients with prominent negative symptoms (including cognitive deficits; Meltzer et al. 1994) compared to classical antipsychotics, which do not increase leptin levels. Reduced motor activity is often present in patients with prominent negative symptoms. Because in contrast to starvation leptin increases motor activity in normal and obese animals (Zhang et al. 1994), one might speculate that an increased, drug-induced leptin production might also contribute to an improvement in motor behavior of patients with schizophrenia.

Conclusions and perspectives

Since its discovery in 1994 the breathtaking research on leptin has yielded, in addition to very strong evidence affirming the important role of leptin in the regulation of food intake, weight and metabolism, growing suspicion that this cytokine-like peptide is also involved in numerous brain functions disturbed in psychiatric patients, such as motor behavior, sleep and cognition. Moreover, like other cytokines, leptin seems to play a role in cell development and survival in both the hematopoietic system and the brain, which is particularly interesting with respect to schizophrenia, a disorder thought to be caused by neurodevelopmental and/or neurodegenerative processes.

The present evidence is sufficient only to conclude that leptin might be involved in the pathophysiology of weight changes occurring in psychiatric disorders, such as anorexia nervosa, and in schizophrenic patients taking drugs that induce weight gain. However, a fine and still incomplete network of data supports speculations that leptin might also be involved in very different symptoms of psychiatric diseases, such as motor behavior in anorexia nervosa and cognition in schizophrenia. Preliminary evidence of reduced leptin production in schizophrenic patients and prominent leptin-enhancing effects of some antipsychotic agents even suggests a future therapeutic role for leptin or newly designed drugs targeting leptin pathways in the treatment of psychiatric disorders.

References

Allison DB, Fontaine KR, Heo M, Mentore JL, Cappelleri JC, Chandler LP, Weiden PJ, Cheskin LJ (1999a) The distribution of body mass index among individuals with and without schizophrenia. J Clin Psychiat 60:215–220

Allison DB, Mentore JL, Heo M, Chandler LP, Cappelleri JC, Infante MC, Weiden PJ (1999b) Antipsychotic-induced weight gain: a comprehensive research synthesis. Am J Psychiat 156:1686–1996

Auwerx J, Staels B (1998) Leptin. Lancet 351:737–742

Beumont PJ, Arthur B, Russell JD, Touyz SW (1994) Excessive physical activity in dieting disorder patients: proposals for a supervised exercise program. Intl J Eat Disord 15:21–36

Brömel T, Blum WF, Ziegler A, Schulz E, Bender M, Fleischhaker C, Remschmidt H, Krieg JC, Hebebrand J (1998) Serum leptin levels increase rapidly after initiation of clozapine therapy. Mol Psychiat 3:76–80

Bukanan R (2000) Schizophrenia: introduction and overview. In: Sadock B, Sadock V (eds) Comprehensive textbook of psychiatry. Lippincott Williams & Wilkins, New York, pp 1096–1109

Bustillo JR, Buchanan RW, Irish D, Breier A (1996) Differential effect of clozapine on weight: a controlled study. Am J Psychiat 153:817–819

Devuyst O, Lambert M, Rodhain J, Lefebvre C, Coche E (1993) Haematological changes and infectious complications in anorexia nervosa: a case-control study. Q J Med 86:791–799

Dicou E, Attoub S, Gressens P (2001) Neuroprotective effects of leptin in vivo and in vitro. Neuroreport 12:3947–3951

Eder U, Mangweth B, Ebenbichler C, Weiss E, Hofer A, Hummer M, Kemmler G, Lechleitner M, Fleischhacker WW (2001) Association of olanzapine-induced weight gain with an increase in body fat. Am J Psychiat 158:1719–1722

Esler M, Vaz M, Collier G, Nestel P, Jennings G, Kaye D, Seals D, Lambert G (1998) Leptin in human plasma is derived in part from the brain, and cleared by the kidneys. Lancet 351(9106):879

Exner C, Hebebrand J, Remschmidt H, Wewetzer C, Ziegler A, Herpertz S, Schweiger U, Blum WF, Preibisch G, Heldmaier G, Klingenspor M (2000) Leptin suppresses semi-starvation induced hyperactivity in rats: implications for anorexia nervosa. Mol Psychiat 5:476–481

Fantuzzi G, Faggioni R (2000) Leptin in the regulation of immunity, inflammation, and hematopoiesis. J Leukocyte Biol 68:437–446

Farooqi IS, Jebb SA, Langmack G, Lawrence E, Cheetham CH, Prentice AM, Hughes IA, McCamish MA, O'Rahilly S (1999) Effects of recombinant leptin therapy in a child with congenital leptin deficiency. N Engl J Med 341:879–884

Hebebrand J, Ballauff A, Hinney A, Herpertz S, Köpp W, Wewetzer C, Ziegler A, Blum WF, Remschmidt H (1999) Die gewichtsregulation im rahmen der Anorexia nervosa unter besonderer berücksichtigung der leptinsekretion. Nervenarzt 70:31–40

Heymsfield SB, Greenberg AS, Fujioka K, Dixon RM, Kushner R, Hunt T, Lubina JA, Patane J, Self B, Hunt P, McCamish M (1999) Recombinant leptin for weight loss in obese and lean adults: a randomized, controlled, dose-escalation trial. JAMA 282:1568–1575

Hinze-Selch D, Schuld A, Kraus T, Kühn M, Uhr M, Haack M, Pollmächer T (2000) Effects of antidepressants on weight and on the plasma levels of leptin, TNF-α and soluble TNF receptors: a longitudinal study in patients treated with amitriptyline or paroxetine. Neuropsychopharmacology 23(1):13–19

Jalenques I, Tauveron I, Albuisson E, Audy V, Fleury-Duhamel N, Codert A (1996) Weight gain as a predictor of long-term clozapine efficiency. Clin Drug Invest 12:16–25

Kalra SP, Dube MG, Pu S, Xu B, Horvath TL, Kalra PS (1999) Interacting appetite-regulating pathways in the hypothalamic regulation of body weight. Endocrine Rev 20:68–100

Karsenty G (2001) Leptin controls bone formation through a hypothalamic relay. Recent Prog Horm Res 56:401–415

Köpp W, Blum WF, von Prittwitz S, Ziegler A, Lubbert H, Emons G, Herzog W, Herpertz S, Deter HC, Remschmidt H, Hebebrand J (1997) Low leptin levels predict amenorrhea in underweight and eating disordered females. Mol Psychiat 2:335–340

Köpp W, Blum WF, Ziegler A, Mathiak K, Lubbert H, Herpertz S, Deter HC, Hebebrand J (1998) Serum leptin and body weight in females with anorexia and bulimia nervosa. Horm Metab Res 30:272–275

Kraepelin E (1901) Einführung in die psychiatrische klinik. Dreissig Vorlesungen. Barth Verlag, Leipzig

Kraus T, Haack M, Schuld A, Hinze-Selch D, Kühn M, Uhr M, Pollmächer T (1999) Body weight and leptin plasma levels during treatment with antipsychotic drugs. Am J Psychiat 156:312–314

Kraus T, Haack M, Schuld A, Hinze-Selch D, Pollmächer T (2001) Low leptin levels but normal body mass indices in patients with depression or schizophrenia. Neuroendocrinology 73:243–247

Kraus T, Zimmermann U, Schuld A, Haack M, Hinze-Selch D, Pollmächer T (2001) Zur patho-physiologie der gewichtsregulation im rahmen der therapie mit Psychopharmaka. Fortschritte der Neurologie-Psychiatrie 69:116–137

Kraus T, Haack M, Schuld A, Hinze-Selch D, Koethe D, Pollmächer T (2002) Body weight, the tumor necrosis factor system and leptin production during treatment with mirtazapine or venlafaxine. Pharmacopsychiatry, in press.

Lieberman JA (1999) Is schizophrenia a neurodegenerative disorder? A clinical and neurobio-logical perspective. Biol Psychiat 46:729–739

Maier W, Lichtermann D, Rietschel M, Held T, Falkai P, Wagner M, Schwab S (1999) [Genetics of schizophrenic disorders. New concepts and findings]. Nervenarzt 70:955–969

Masuzaki H, Ogawa Y, Hosoda K, Miyawaki T, Hanaoka I, Hiraoka J, Yasuno A, Nishimura H, Yoshimasa Y, Nishi S, Nakao K (1997) Glucocorticoid regulation of leptin synthesis and secretion in humans: elevated plasma leptin levels in Cushing's syndrome. J Clin Endocrin Metab 82:2542–2547

Meltzer HY, Lee MA, Ranjan R (1994) Recent advances in the pharmacotherapy of schizophre-nia. Acta Psychiatr Scand 384:95–101

Morimoto T, Yamamoto Y, Yamatodani A (2001) Brain histamine and feeding behavior. Behav Brain Res 124:145–150

Newcomer JW, Selke G, Melson AK, Gross J, Vogler GP, Dagogo-Jack S (1998) Dose-dependent cortisol-induced increases in plasma leptin concentration in healthy humans. Arch Gen Psy-chiat 55:995–1000

Pickar D (1995) Prospects for pharmacotherapy of schizophrenia. Lancet 345:557–562

Pollmächer T (2002) Treatment of schizophrenia. In: Smelser NJ, Balters PB (eds) International Encyclopedia of the social and behavioral sciences. Pergamon, Kidlington, pp 13546–13552

Rayner DV, Trayhurn P (2001) Regulation of leptin production: sympathetic nervous system interactions. J Mol Med 79:8–20

Schafroth U, Godang K, Ueland T, Bollerslev J (2001) Leptin response to endogenous acute stress is independent of pituitary function. Eur J Endocrinol 145:295–301

Shanley LJ, Irving AJ, Harvey J (2001) Leptin enhances NMDA receptor function and modulates hippocampal synaptic plasticity. J Neuroscience 21(24):RC186

Sinton CM, Fitch TE, Gershenfeld HK (1999) The effects of leptin on REM sleep and slow wave delta in rats are reversed by food deprivation. J Sleep Res 8:197–203

Steppan CM, Swick AG (1999) A role for leptin in brain development. Biochem Biophys Res Commun 256:600–602

Wauters M, Considine RV, Van Gaal LF (2000) Human leptin: from an adipocyte hormone to an endocrine mediator. Eur J Endocrinol 143:293–311

Zhang Y, Proenca R, Maffei M, Barone M, Leopold L, Friedman JM (1994) Positional cloning of the mouse obese gene and its human homologue. Nature 372:425–432

Genomic approach to common human obesity

P. Boutini[1] and P. Froguel[1,2]

Summary

Obesity is a typical, common, multifactorial disease in that environmental and genetic factors interact. Environmental risk factors like unlimited access to food apply constant pressure in subjects with a genetic predisposition to gain weight. The identification of different monogenic forms of human obesity [mutations of the leptin gene and its receptor, proopiomelenocortine (POMC), prohormone convertase 1 (PC1) in the melanocortin receptor 4 (MC4R)] established that genetic defects can cause human obesity. The more common forms of obesity are, however, polygenic. To date, two general approaches have been taken in the search for genes underlying common polygenic obesity in human. The first approach focused on genes selected as having some plausible role in obesity, on the basis of their known or presumed biological role. This approach only yielded putative susceptibility genes with a small or uncertain effect. The second approach attempted to map genes purely by position and required no presumptions about the function of the genes. Genome-wide scans identified chromosomal regions showing linkage with obesity in large collections of nuclear families. Genome-wide scans in different ethnic populations localized major obesity loci on chromosomes 2, 4, 5, 7, 10, 11 and 20. Susceptibility gene(s) for obesity may be positionally cloned in the intervals of linkage. The systematic use of SNPs markers for linkage disequilibrium mapping strategy combined with functional genomics will be helpful in better understanding the molecular determinants of obesity.

The candidate-gene approach and the positional cloning of major obesity-linked regions approach are discussed in this paper

Introduction

Obesity is a common disease that has become more prevalent in all countries over the past few years (Wordl Health Organization 1997). About 8 to 10 % of the French population, 17 to 20 % in England and Wales and over 25 % of North Americans are obese [Wordl Health Organization 1997; Maillard et al. 2000; Prescott-Clarke and primatesta 1998). In Europe, although obesity is less preva-

---

[1]CNRS-Institute of Biology of Lille, Pasteur Institute of Lille, France
[2]Barts and The London Genome Centre, London, UK

Kordon et al.
Brain Somatic Cross-Talk and the
Central Control of Metabolism
© Springer-Verlag Berlin Heidelberg 2002

lent in adults than in the U.S., the prevalence of overweight is increasing among children and teenagers. In France, latest data showed that 16 % of children and teenagers are overweight and the number of obese children had multipled by five in the last 10 years (Maillard et al. 2000). Obesity is a risk factor for early mortality and a wide range of metabolic and cardiovascular complications (Lean et al. 1998).

Although rapid globalisation of the westernised way of life is responsible for the outstanding rise in numbers of obesity cases (about 1 billion subjects are now overweight or frankly obese), obesity is a typical, common, multifactorial disease in that environmental and genetic factors interact, resulting in a disease state (Bouchard 1991). There is strong evidence for a genetic component to human obesity, e.g., the familial clustering (relative risk among sibs of 3 to 7; Allison et al. 1996), and the high concordance of body composition in monozygotic twins (Maes et al. 1997). However, the role of genetic factors in common obesity is complex, being determined by interaction of several genes (polygenic), each of which may have relatively small effects (i.e., they are susceptibility genes) and work in combination with each other as well as with environmental factors (such as nutrients, physical activity, smoking). As complex traits arise through the concerted action of multiple genetic factors (through a network implying genetic heterogeneity and epistatic interactions) with different and strong environmental factors, the task of identifying any single susceptibility factor is problematic.

In monogenic obesity, the candidat-gene approach identified five different causative genes: leptin gene and its receptor, proopiomelenocortine (POMC), prohormone convertase 1 (PC1) and the melanocortin receptor 4 (MC4R; Montague et al. 1997; Clement et al. 1998; Krude et al. 1998; Vaisse et al. 1998; Yeo et al. 1998; Jackson et al. 1997). All these obesity gene-encoded proteins are connected in the same leptin pathway for weight control. In contrast, the genetic approach of polygenic obesity has been less successful to date. Despite many claims, most of the investigated genes failed to provide convincing and unambiguous evidence of involvement in the genetic risk for obesity. The Reasons are numerous, with one of the most important being the weakness of our knowledge of the molecular mechanisms of energy balance, and another being the frequent lack of well-conducted studies of candidate genes in large populations with reliable phenotypes. Two general approaches (candidate-genes and genome-wide scans) have been conducted to date in the search for genes underlying common polygenic obesity in humans.

Candidate-gene approach

Candidate genes are selected as having some plausible role in obesity, based on their known or presumed biological role in energy homeostasis. Efforts to identify candidate genes for obesity have concentrated on adipose tissue. In brown adipose tissue, regulation of thermogenesis by the sympathetic nervous system is mediated by beta adrenergic receptors (Nonogaki 2000). In humans, Beta-3 adrenergic receptors (beta3-AR) are modestly expressed in fat and adipocytes lining the gastrointestinal tract (Krief et al. 1993). A Trp64Arg mutation located in

the first transmembrane domain of the receptor was first identified as being correlated with obesity in Pima Indians, Frenchmen and Finns (Walston et al. 1995;
Clement et al. 1995; Widen et al. 1995). However, discordant association as well as
functional studies were also published (Buettner et al. 1998; Chosh et al. 1999), indicating that the role of this candidate gene in human obesity, if any, is modest or
should be considered in relation with others in the same pathway. Importantly, in
mature brown adipocyte cells, stimulation of beta3-AR by norepinephrine activates uncoupling protein 1 (UCP-1) via the cAMP metabolic pathway. Uncoupling
proteins (UCPs) are inner mitochondrial membrane transporters that dissipates
the proton gradient, releasing stored energy in the form of heat (Klingenberger
1990). An A to G variation in UCP-1 is associated with a gain of fat mass in a Quebec family study (Oppert et al. 1994). Additional effects of the G allele of the -3826
variant of UCP1 with the Trp64Arg mutation of beta3-AR gene occurred in the
French morbid obese population (Klement et al. 1996). Recently, synergic effects
UCP1 with beta3AR polymorphism in decreasing sympathetic nervous system
activity were observed in a Japanese populatio (Shihara et al. 2001). Polymorphisms in other members of the uncoupling gene families, UCP2 and UCP3, are
associated with BMI in Pima Indians (Walder et al. 1998). In addition, a common
polymorphism in the promoter of UCP2 is associated with enhanced mRNA expression and decreased risk of obesity (Esterbauer et al. 2001). Recent data from a
UCP2 KO mice (Arsenijevic et al. 2000) showed no effect on body weight. In contrast, there is now evidence that UCP2 is a potent inhibitor of insulin secretion,
these UCP2 KO mice exhibit hyperinsulinemia. All these uncertainties illustrate
the complexity of the candidate-gene approach, especially when gene function is
not perfectly known.

Several other candidate genes have been studied for the presence of an association with BMI, body fat and other obesity-related phenotypes and they are reported annually in a review paper in *Obi Research* (Rankinen et al. 2002). Unfortunately, the candidate-gene approach has, to date, only yielded putative susceptibility genes with a small or uncertain effect. This lack of power could be explained by the restricted choice of candidates, due to our ignorance of disturbed
pathways in the excess of fat storage. However, extensive gene-targeting experiments mice and functional genomics (expression profiles in different tissues of
interest for energy balance), together with the near completion of the Human
Genome Project have provided a new generation of candidate genes for obesity.
The choice of an ideal candidate gene may be based on several criteria, including
its chromosomal localisation (obesity–linked locus inhuman or in animal models), its expression profile (i.e., in adipocyte or in hypothalamus), and its expression, regulated by food intake, nutrients or by physical activity.

Genome-wide scan approach

The genome-wide scan strategy requires no presumptions about the function of
genes at the susceptibility loci, since it attempts to map genes purely by position
and by detecting chromosomal regions showing linkage with obesity in large collections of nuclear families. Genotyping of 400 multiallelic markers [short tan-

dem repeats (STRs) with a density of 1 marker/10cM] enables identification of polymorphic markers showing strong allele identity by descent in obese family members (i.e., allele sharing in sibships is significantly higher than 50 %). Identification of such susceptibility gene(s) for obesity may then be positionally cloned in the intervals of linkage.

Genome-wide scans for obesity genes have been carried out in Mexican-American families(Comuzzie et al. 1997), French pedigrees (Hager et al. 1998), Pima Indians (Norman et al. 1997; Hanson et al. 1998), and in white Americans (Lee et al. 1999; Kissebah et al. 2000; Stone et al. 2002; Rice et al. 2002; Feitosa et al. 2002). Both Comuzzie et al. (1997) and Hager et al. (1998) provided a candidate region on chromosome 2p21 that could explain a significant part of the variance of leptin levels in human. This linkage was replicated in a cohort of African-American families (Rotimi et al. 1999). Other major genes loci for obesity and leptin levels were identified on chromosome 10p11 and on 5cen-q in French families. This 10p locus may account for 20–30 % of the genetic risk for obesity in this population (Hager et al. 1998). The involvement of this chromosomal region in obesity was recently confirmed in a cohort of young obese German (Hinney et al. 2000), as well as in White Caucasians, African Americans (Price et al. 2001), and the old-order Amish (Hsueh et al. 2001). In addition to this 10p locus, a genome scan performed in white Americans showed evidence for linkage on chromosome 20q 13 and on 10q (Lee et al. 1999). In Pima Indians, the most interesting region was shown on chromosome 11q (Norman et al. 1997). Recently, Comuzzie described a new locus at 3q27 that was linked to various quantitative traits characterizing the metabolic/insulin resistance syndrome (Kisebah et al. 2000). Interestingly, this 3q27 locusl was previously identified as a T2DM locus in the French population (Vionnet et al. 2000). Several candidate genes map to this region, including the APM1 gene encoding the differentiated adipocyte secreted protein ACRP30/adiponectin, which is abundantly present in plasma. The purified C-terminal domain of adiponectin has been reported to protect mice on a high fat diet from obesity and to rescue obese or lipoatropic mouse models from severe insulin resistance, by decreasing levels of plasma free fatty acids (FFA) and enhancing lipid oxidization in muscle (Fruebis et al. 2001). Moreover, plasma levels of adiponectin have been shown to be decreased in obese diabetic subjects (Arita et al. 1999, and decreased adiponectin is implicated in the development of insulin resistance in mouse models of both obesity and lipoatrophy (Yamamuchi et al. 2001), which makes ACRP30 an attractive candidate gene for fat-induced metabolic syndrome and T2DM. Genetic variation in the gene encoding adiponectin is associated with an increased risk of type 2 diabetes in the Japanese population (Hara et al. 2002). A recent study suggests that an at-risk haplotype of common variants of ACRP30 located in the promoter and rare mutations in exon 3 contribute to the variation of the adipocyte-secreted adiponectin hormone level and may be part of the genetic determinants for T2D in the French Caucasian population (Vasseur et al. 2002).

Although some concerns have been raised about the heterogeneity and reliability of genetic data in multifactorial diseases in general (e.g., the lack of replication), Genome-wide scan studies suggest that, among complex traits, adiposity is one of the most inheritable, and that few major loci may contribute to the genetic risk for obesity in human. A working hypothesis based on available data is that obesity is an oligogenic disease whose development can be modulated by various polygenic (modifier genes) and environmental influences.

Positional cloning strategy: Towards the identification of common obesity genes

To identify the true etiological gene variants associated with the enhanced risk for "typical" overweight, chromosomal regions of linkage shoufd first be refined using a dense map of biallelic single-nucleotide polymorphisms (SNPs). Indeed, the state of the art in positional cloning of complex disorder susceptibility genes implies that the systematic use of SNPs markers can be useful for the detection of linkage disequilibrium mapping (LD mapping; Terwilliger and Weiss 1998; Zollner et al., Abecasis et al. 2001). Indeed, DNA polymorphisms located away from the true functional variant can be associated with obesity or with the variation of an obesity associated trait. The strength of LD is quite variable within the genome, ranging from 10 Kb to 300 Kb or more. It had been postulated that working in a so-called "isolated" population would significantly increase LD expectancy, but recent evidence showed that even working in Finns or in Icelanders is not a panacea (Eaves et al. 2000). The recent identification of the NIDDMI gene (calpain 10) on 2q confirmed that LD mapping could be a successful strategy for unravelling other polygenic diseases (Horikawa et al. 2000). However, this work also showed the complexity of the search, as, in this case, an intronic polymorphism (UCSNP-43) was associated with type 2 diabetes in Mexican Americans. In fact, three non-coding polymorphisms, including UCSNP-43, have been identified defining an at-risk haplotype. In other ethnic groups, like French Caucasians, the rarity of this high-risk haplotype makes difficult a definite answer about the role of calpain 10 in T2D. Moreover, as the function of this protease is still unclear, this study has emphasised the limitation of genetic studies to prove a functional relation from solely statistic-based methods.

Conclusion

Genetic and functional studies in humans will be associated in synergy with LD mapping strategy. For example, tissue profiling may provide the most direct way to improve overall understanding of the molecular circuitry maintaining energy homeostasis. Therefore, expression profiling in humans on one hand and genetic analysis of populations on the other hand will provide complementary tools to advance our understanding of the complex network of gene-gene and gene-environment interactions underlying the susceptibility to obesity. Following identification of genetic variations, the exploration of the consequences at the tissue (tissue profiling), organism and population (molecular epidemiology) levels will clarify the role of these variants in the disease pathogenesis and their implications for diagnostic and therapeutic developments. Recent studies in patients with prostate cancer (Tartiglian et al. 2001), inflammatory bowel disease (Hugot et al. 2001), and psoriasis (Asumalahti et al 2002). show evidence of the resolution of linkage to identify a candidate gene. Improved understanding of genetic and environmental predictors of risk factors provides a rational basis for stratification of the disease risk and the response to treatment, allowing effective targeting of preventive and therapeutic tools.

References

Abecasis GR, Noguchi E, Heinzmann A, Traherne JA, Bhattacharyya S, Leaves NI, Anderson GG, Zhang Y, Lench NJ, Carey A, Cardon LR, Moffatt MF, Cookson WO (2001) Extent and distribution of linkage Disequilibrium in Three Genomic Regions. Am J Human Genet 68(1):191–197

Allison DB, Faith MS, Nathan JS (1996) Risch's lambda values for human obesity. Intl J Obesity 20:990–999

Arita Y, Kihara S, Ouchi N, Takahashi M, Maeda K, Miyagawa J, Hotta K, Shimomura I, Nakamura T, Miyaoka K, Kuriyama H, Nishida M, Yamashita S, Okubo K, Matsubara K, Muraguchi M, Ohmoto Y, Funahashi T, Matsubwa Y (1999) Paradoxical decrease of an adipose-specific protein, adiponectin, in obesity. Biochem Biophys Res Commun 257:79–83

Arsenijevic D, Onuma H, Pecqueur C, Raimbault S, Manning BS, Miroux B, Couplan E, Alves-Guerra MC, Goubem M, Surwit R, Bouillaud F, Richard D, Collins S, Ricquier D (2000) Disruption of the uncoupling protein-2 gene in mice reveals a role in immunity reactive oxygen species production. Nature Genet 26:435–439

Asumalahti K, Veal C, Laitinen T, Suomela S, Allen M, Elomaa O, Moser M, de Cid R, Ripatti S, Vorechovsky I, Marcusson JA, Nakagawa H, Lazaro C, Estivill X, Capon F, Novelli G, Saarialho-Kere U, Barker J, Trembath R, Kere J (2002) Coding haplotype analysis supports HCR as the putative susceptibility gene for psoriasis at the MHC PSORS1 locus. Human Mol Genet 11(5):589–597

Bouchard C (1991) Current understanding of aetiology of obesity genetic and non genetic factors. Am J Clin Nutri 53:1561–1565

Buettner R, Schaffler A, Arndt H, Rogler G, Nusser J, Zietz B, Enger I, Hugl S, Cuk A, Scholmerich J, Palitzsch KD (1998) The Trp64Arg polymorphism of the beta3adrenergic receptor gene is not associated with obesity or type 2 diabetes mellitus in a large population-based caucasian cohort. J Clin Endocrinol Meta 83(11):2892–2897

Clement K, Ruiz J, Cassard-Doulcier AM, Bouillaud F, Ricquier D, Basdevant A, Guy-Grand B, Froguel P (1996) Additive effects of polymorphims in the uncoupling protein gene and the beta-3 adrenergic receptor gene on gain weight in morbid obesity. Int J Obesity 20:1062–1066

Clement K, Vaisse C, Lahlou N, Cabrol S, Pelloux V, Cassuto D, Gourmelen M, Dina C, Chambaz J, Lacorte JM, Basdevant A, Bougneres P, Lebouc Y, Froguel P, Guy GB (1998) A mutation in the human leptin receptor gene causes obesity and pituitary dysfunction. Nature 392:398–401

Clement K, Vaisse C, Manning BS, Basdevant A, Guy-Grand B, Ruiz J, Silver KD, Shuldiner AR, Froguel P, Strosberg AD (1995) Genetic variation in the beta 3 adrenergic

Comuzzie AG, Hixson JE, Almasy L, Mitchell BD, Mahaney MC, Dyer TD, Stern MP, MacCluer JW, Blangero J (1997) A major quantitative trait locus determining serum leptin levels and fat mass is located on human chromosome 2. Nature Genet 15(3):273–276

Eaves IA, Merriman TR, Barber RA, Nutland S, Tuomilehto-Wolf E, Tuomilehto J, Cucca F, Todd JA (2000) The genetically isolated populations of Finland and Sardinia may not be a panacea for linkage disequilibrium mapping of common disease genes. Nature Genet 25:320–323

Esterbauer H, Schneider C, Oberkoffer H, Ebenbichler C, Paulweber B, Sandhofer F, Ladumer G, Hell E, Strosberg AD, Patsch JR, Krempler F, Patsch W (2001) A common polymorphism in the promoter of UCP2 is associated with decreased risk of obesity in middle-aged humans. Nature Genet 28:178–183

Feitosa MF, Borecki IB, Rich SS, Arnett DK, Sholinsky P, Myers RH, Leppert M, Province MA (2002) Quantitative trait loci influencing body-mass index reside on chromosomes 7 and 13: The National Heart Lung and Blood Institute family heart study. Am J Human Genet 70:72–82

Fruebis J, Tsao TS, Javorschi S, Ebbets-Reed D, Erickson MR, Yen FT, Bihain BE, Lodish HF (2001) Proteolytic cleavage product of 30-kDa adipocyte complement-related protein increases fatty acid oxidation in muscle and causes weight loss in mice. Proc Nat Acad Sci USA 98:2005–2010

Ghosh S, Langefeld CD, Ally D, Watanabe RM, Hauser ER, Magnuson VL, Nylund SJ, Valle T, Eriksson J, Bergman RN, Tuomilehto J, Collins FS, Boehnke M (1999) The W64R variant of the beta3-adrenergic receptor gene is not associated with type 2 diabetes or obesity in a large Finnish sample. Diabetologia 42(2):238–244

Hager J, Dina C, Francke S, Dubois S, Houari M, Vatin V, Vaillant E, Lorentz N, Basdevant A, Clement K, Guy-Grand B, Froguel P (1998) A genome-wide scan for human obesity genes shows evidence for a major susceptibility locus on chromosome 10. Nature Genet 20:304–338

Hanson RL, Ehm MG, Pettitt DJ, Prochazka M, Thompson DB, Timberlake D, Foroud T, Kobes S, Baier L, Burns DK, Almasy L, Blangero J, Garvey WT, Bennett PH, Knowler WC (1998) An autosomal genomic scan for loci linked to type II diabetes mellitus and body-mass index in Pima Indians. Am J Human Genet 63:1130–1138

Hara K, Boutin P, Mori Y, Tobe K, Dina C, Yasuda K, Yamauchi T, Otabe S,Okada T, Eto K,Kadowaki H, Hagura R, Akanuma Y, Yazaki Y, Nagai R, Taniyama M, Matsubara K, Yoda M, Nakano Y, Tomita M, Kimura S, Ito C, Froguel P, Kadowaki T (2002) Genetic variation in the gene encoding adiponectin is associated with an increased risk of type 2 diabetes in the Japanese population. Diabetes 51(4):1294

Hinney A, Ziegler A, Oeffner F, Wedewardt C, Vogel M, Wulftange H, Geller F, Stubing K, Siegfried W, Goldschmidt HP, Remschmidt H, Hedebrand J (2000) Independant confirmation of a major locus for obesity on chromosome 10. J Clin Endocrinol Metab 85(8):2962–2965

Horikawa Y, Oda N, Cox NJ, Li X, Orho-Melander M, Hara M, Hinokio Y, Lindner TH, Mashima H, Schwarz PE, del Bosque-Plata L, Horikawa Y, Oda Y,Yoshiuchi I, Colilla S, Polonsky KS, Wei S, Concannon P, Iwasaki N, Schulze J, Baier LJ, Bogardus C, Groop L, Boerwinkle E, Hanis CL, Bell GI (2000) Genetic variation in the gene encoding calpain-10 is associated with type 2 diabetes mellitus. Nature Genet 26:163–175

Hsueh WC, Mitchell BD, Schneider JL, St Jean PL, Pollin TI, Ehm MG, Wagner MJ, Burns DK, Sakul H, Bell CJ, Shuldiner AR (2001) Genome-wide scan of obesity in the old order Amish. The J Clin Endocrinol Metab 86(3):1199–1205

Hugot JP, Chamaillard M, Zouali H, Lesage S, Cezard JP, Belaiche J, Almer S, Tysk C, O'Morain CA, Gassull M, Binder V, Finkel Y, Cortot A, Modigliani R, Laurent-Puig P, Gower-Rousseau C, Macry J, Colombel JF, Sahbatou M, Thomas G (2001) Association of NOD2 leucine-rich repeat variants with susceptibility to Crohn's disease. Nature 31(411):599–603

Jackson RS, Creemers JW, Ohagi S, Raffin-Sanson ML, Sanders L, Montague CT, Hutton JC, O'Rahilly S (1997) Obesity and impaired prohormone processing associated with mutations in the human prohormone convertase 1 gene. Nature Genet 16:303–306

Kissebah AH, Sonnenberg GE, Myklebust J, Goldstein M, Broman K, James RG, Marks JA, Krakower GR, Jacob HJ,Weber J, Martin L, Blangero J, Comuzzie AG (2000) Quantitative trait loci on chromosome 3 and 17 influence phenotypes of the metabolic syndrome. Proc Nat Acad Sci USA 97:14478–14483

Klingenberger M (1990) Mechanism and evolution of the uncoupling protein of brown adipose tissue. Trends Biochem Sci 15:108–112

Krief S, Lonnqvist F, Raimbault S, Baude B, Van Spronsen A, Amer P, Strosberg AD, Ricquier D, Emorine LJ (1993) Tissue distribution of beta3-adrenergic receptor nRNA in man. J Clini Investi 91:344–349

Krude H, Biebermann H, Luck W, Horn R, Brabant G, Gruters A (1998) Severe early-onset obesity, adrenal insufficiency and red hair pigmentation caused by POMC mutations in humans. Nature Genet 19(2):155–157

Lee JH, Reed DR, Li WD, Xu W, Joo EJ, Kilker RL, Nanthakumar E, North M, Sakul H, Bell C, Price RA (1999) Genome scan for human obesity and linkage to markers in 20q13. Am J Human Genet 64(1):196–209

Maes HH, Neale MC, Eaves LJ (1997) Genetic and environmental factors in relative body weight and human adiposity. Behav Genet 27:325–351

Maillard G, Charles MA, Thibult N, Forhan A, Sermet C, Basdevant A, Eschwege E (2000) Trends in the prevalence of obesity in children and adolescents in France between 1980 and 1991. Intl J Obesity 24(12):1608–1617

Montague CT, Farooqi IS, Whitehead JP, Soos MA, Rau H, Wareham NJ, Sewter CP, Digby JE, Mohammed SN, Hurst JA, Cheetham CH, Earley AR, Barnett AH, Prins JB, O'Rahilly S (1997) Congenital leptin deficiency is associated with severe early-onset obesity in humans. Nature 387:903–908

Nonogaki K (2000) New insights into sympathetic regulation of glucose and fat metabolism. Diabetologia 43:533–549

Norman RA, Thompson DB, Foroud T, Garvey WT, Bennett PH, Bogardus C, Ravussin E (1997) Genomewide search for genes influencing percent body fat in Pima Indians : suggestive linkage at chromosome 11q21–q22. Am J Human Genet 60:166–173

Oppert JM, Vohl MC, Chagnon M, Dionne FT, Cassard-Doulcier AM, Ricquier D, Perusse L, Bouchard C (1994) DNA polymorphism in the uncoupling protein (UCP) gene and human body fat. Int J Obesity 18:526–531

Prescott-Clarke P, Primatesta P (1996) Health survey for England HMSO, London Lean MEJ, Hans TS, Seidell JC (1998) Impairment of health and quality life in people with large waist circumference. Lancet 351: 853–856

Price RA, Li WD, Bernstein A, Crystal A, Golding EM, Weisberg SJ, Zuckerman WA (2001) A locus affecting obesity in human chromosome region 10p12. Diabetologia 44363–366

Rankinen T, Perusse L, Weisnagel SJ, Snyder EE, Chagnon YC, Bouchard C (2002) The human obesity gene map : The 2001 update. Obesity Res 10(3):196–243

receptor gene and an increased capacity to gain weight in patients with morbid obesity. New Engl J Med 333:352–354

Rice T, Chagnon YC, Perusse L, Borecki IB, Ukkola O, Rankinen T, Gagnon J, Leon AS, Skinner JS, Wilmore JH, Bouchard C, Rao DC (2002) A genomewide linkage scan for abdominal subcutaneous and visceral fat in black and white families: The HERITAGE family study. Diabetes 51(3):848–855

Rotimi CN, Comuzzie AG, Lowe WL, Luke A, Blangero J, Cooper RS (1999) The quantitative trait locus on chromosome 2 for serum leptin levels is confirmed in African-Americans. Diabetes 48:643–644

Shihara N, Yasuda K, Moritani T, Ue H, Uno M, Adachi T, Nunoi K, Seino Y, Yamada Y, Tsuda K (2001) Synergic effect of polymorphisms of uncoupling proteinl and beta3-adrenergic receptor genes on autonomic nervous system activity. Int J Obesity Related Metab Disord 25(6):761–766

Single Nucleotide Polymorphism haplotypes in the both proximal promoter and exon 3 of APM1 gene modulate adipocyte-secreted adiponectin hormone levels and contribute to the genetic risk for Type 2 Diabetes in French Caucasians. Human Mol Genet

Stone S, Abkevich V, Hunt SC, Gutin A, Russell DL, Neff CD, Riley R, Frech GC, Hensel CH, Jammulapati S, Potter J, Sexton D, Tran T, Gibbs D, Iliev D, Gress R, Bloomquist B, Amatruda J, Rae PM, Adams TD, Skolnick MH, Shattuck D (2002) A major Predisposition locus for severe obesity, at 4p15–p14. Am J Human Genet 70(6):1459–6836

Tavtigian SV, Simard J, Teng DH, Abtin V, Baumgard M, Beck A, Camp NJ, Carillo AR, Chen Y, Dayananth P, Desrochers M, Dumont M, Farnham JM, Frank D, Frye C, Ghaffari S, Gupte JS, Hu R, Iliev D, Janecki T, Kort EN, Laity KE, Leavitt A, Leblanc G, McArthur-Morrison J, Pederson A, Penn B, Peterson KT, Reid JE, Richards S, Schroeder M, Smith R, Snyder SC, Swedlund B, Swensen J, Thomas A, Tranchant M, Woodland AM, Labrie F, Skolnick MH, Neuhausen S, Rommens J, Cannon-Albright LA (2001) A candidate prostate cancer susceptibility gene at chromosome 17p. Nature Genet 27:172–180

Terwilliger JD, Weiss KM (1998) Linkage disequilibrium mapping of complex disease: fantasy or reality? Curr Opin Biotechnol 9:578–594

Vaisse C, Clement K, Guy GB, Froguel P (1998) A frameshift mutation in human MC4R is associated with a dominant form of obesity. Nature Genet 20:113–114

Vasseur F, Helbecque N, Dina C, Lobbens S, Delannoy V, Gaget S, Boutin P, Vaxillaire M, Leprêtre F, Dupont S, Hara K, Clément K, Kadowaki T, Froguel P (2002)

Vionnet N, Hani El-H, Dupont S, Gallina S, Francke S, Dotte S, De Matos F, Durand E, Lepretre F, Lecoeur C, Gallina P, Zekiri L, Dina C, Froguel P (2000) Genomewide search for type 2 diabetes-susceptibility genes in french whites : evidence for a novel susceptibility locus for early-onset diabetes on chromosome 3q27-qter and independant replication of a type 2-diabetes locus on chromosome 1q21–q24. Am J Human Genet 67:1470–1480

Walder K, Norman RA, Hanson RL, Schrauwen P, Neverova M, Jenkinson CP, Easlick J, Warden CH, Pecqueur C, Raimbault S, Ricquier D, Silver MH, Shuldiner AR, Solanes G, Lowell BB, Chung WK, Leibel RL, Pratley R, Ravussin E (1998) Association between uncoupling protein polymorphisms (UCP2–UCP3) and energy metabolism obesity in Pima Indians. Human Mol Genet 7:1431–1435

Walston J, Silver K, Bogardus C, Knowler WC, Celi FS, Austin S, Manning B, Strosberg AD, Stern MP, Raben N, Sorkin JD, Roth J, Shuldiner AR (1995) Time of onset of non-insulin dependant diabetes mellitus and genetic variation in the beta3adrenergic receptor gene. New Engl J Med 333:343–348

Widen WE, Lehto M, Kanninen T, Walston J, Shuldiner AR, Groop LC (1995) Association of a polymorphism in the beta3-adrenergic receptor gene with features of the insulin resistance syndrome in Finns. New Engl J Med 333:348–352

World Health Organization (1997) Obesity: preventing and managing the global epidemic. Report of a WHO consultation on Obesity. Geneva, 3–5 June 1997

Yamauchi T, Kamon J, Waki H, Terauchi Y, Kubota N, Hara K, Mori Y, Ide T, Murakami K, Tsuboyama-Kasaoka N, Ezaki O, Akanuma Y, Gavrilova O, Vinson C, Reitman ML, Kagechika H, Shudo K, Yoda M, Nakano Y, Tobe K, Nagai R, Kimura S, Tomita M, Froguel P, Kadowaki T (2001) The fat-derived hormone adiponectin reverses insulin resistance associated with both lipoatrophy and obesity. Nature Med 7(8):941–946

Yeo GS, Farooqi IS, Aminian S, Halsall DJ, Stanhope RG, O'Rahilly S (1998) A frameshift mutation in MC4R associated with dominantly inherited human obesity. Nature Genet 20(2):111–112

Zollner S, Von Haeseler A (2000) A coalescent approach to study linkage disequilibrium between single-nucleotide polymorphisms. Am J Human Genet 66:615–628

The Epigenetic Inheritance Hypothesis

C. Junien[1]

Evolution according to Lamarck and Darwin

At the beginning of the 19th century, long before the work of Charles Darwin (1809–1882), whose theory of evolution (slow; "The Origin of Species" 1859) by natural selection has been accepted for over a century, Jean-Baptiste Lamarck (1744–1829) suggested that species vary and introduced the concept of evolution. These two scientists played an important role in the discovery of the mechanisms of evolution. Jean-Baptiste Lamarck seems to be the real founder of the theory of evolution of living beings: this French naturalist first stated that life could appear at any moment, as a result of spontaneous generation from inanimate sources. He then proposed that primitive organisms (which he called infusoria) form themselves into increasingly complex organisms. According to Lamarck, there are two reasons why species evolve towards more and more sophisticated forms: the spontaneous tendency of living material to move towards perfection and, secondly, the effect of the environment. Adaptation to the environment modifies an organism's needs, creating new habits that in turn lead to changes in the organism. Thus, according to Lamarck, the use or lack of use of an organ leads to the development or degeneration of that organ. Based on this theory, Lamarck stated that the characteristics acquired by a generation are transmitted, via heredity, to the following generations. This latter point was finally the most contested. It is summarised in Lamarck's fourth law, regarding the organisation of individuals (1816): *"All traits that are acquired, traced or changed in the organisation of individuals, during the course of their life, are conserved by that generation and transmitted to their offspring"* (Fig. 1).

This idea that certain characteristics are almost systematically, directly transmitted from one generation to the next long appeared to be contrary to the slowness of the evolution of species. In contrast, Darwin described a process much closer to reality in which genetic characteristics were transmitted over time (if only since the appearance of the first hominids six to eight million years ago!). However, if we consider Lamarck's fourth law in terms of epigenetic processes or adaptive mechanisms controlled by stress proteins and transposable sequences, rather than in genetic terms, it may be possible to conciliate the theories of Darwin and Lamarck.

---

[1] Inserm U383 "Génétique, Chromosome et Cancer", Université Paris V, Hôpital Necker – Enfants Malades, 149 Rue de Sèvres, 75015 Paris

Kordon et al.
Brain Somatic Cross-Talk and the
Central Control of Metabolism
© Springer-Verlag Berlin Heidelberg 2002

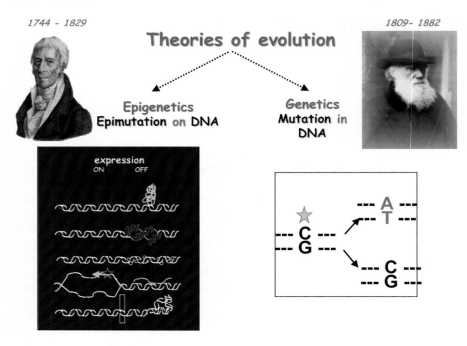

Fig. 1. Lamarck and Darwin: genetics and epigenetics. Although the archetypal Lamarckian fourth law is clearly wrong, there are indeed some characteristics that are affected by random heritable epimutations (epi = on, in Greek), mutations that do not affect the DNA sequence itself. There is a surprising degree of phenotypic variation among genetically identical individuals, even when the environmental influences are identical. This intangible variation results from the stochastic establishement of epigenetic modifications to the DNA nucleotide sequence. These modifications, which may involve cytosine methylation and chromatin remodelling, result in alteration in gene expression, which in turn affects the phenotype of the organism. In contrast with these epimutations, which do not alter the DNA sequence and can be reversible, the classical Mendelian mutations that are required for a Darwinian type of evolution under selective pressure require a change in DNA sequence involving one or several base changes in the nucleotide sequence. An epimutation does not modify the nucleotide sequence but leads to changes in the behaviour (abolition or reduction of expression, or activation of expression) of this sequence due to methylation, chromatin condensation, the binding of protein factors or the acetylation of histones. The genomes of many species are compartmentalised with various degrees of compaction. The transcriptionally active regions consist of a more relaxed chromatin, whereas the transcriptionally inactive regions and heterochromatin regions are highly condensed and not very accessible to transcription factors. DNA methylation is one of the processes involved in the assembly of chromatin. Chromatin is formed from chains of nucleosomes, each containing 180 to 200 base pairs of DNA wrapped around histones. Acetylated histones are usually rich in transcription-competent chromatin, whereas transcriptionally inactive chromatin is usually deacetylated and, in some cases, methylated. Classical mutations and epimutations affecting the somatic line are not transmitted, unless they occur at an early stage, before the differentiation of the two lines. Like classical mutations, only epimutations that affect the germline can be transmitted to the next generation.

Dietary habits have always fluctuated

Excess weight and obesity are becoming more common in industrialised countries and in developing countries. They are known risk factors for glucose intolerance, insulin resistance and type 2 diabetes with hyperlipidaemia, hypertension and increased cardiovascular risk. Major changes in the dietary habits of humans (excess protein and energy) and a more sedentary lifestyle are probably at the origin of an increase in the fat content of the body due to an imbalance between energy intake and expenditure. Other qualitative factors are also involved, as obesity is especially common in poorer populations. These environmental changes have so far affected two to three generations and it is difficult to estimate how future generations will adapt in the long term to this new environment.

Man's relationship with his food has changed dramatically between prehistoric times, when fire was first mastered, and the present day. Our ancestors were hunters and tended to be more carnivorous. They ate far more animal fats and proteins than the sedentary humans that succeeded them in Neolithic times. This type of food enabled them to survive in extremely difficult conditions. Dramatic changes occurred with the development of animal husbandry and agriculture about ten to twelve thousand years ago. As humans became more sedentary, food became much richer in carbohydrates, and domesticated animals provided milk. The development of agriculture led to the consumption of a diet essentially composed of agricultural products. More recently, in 1791, the chemist and nutritionist Lavoisier reviewed the "territorial richness of the kingdom of France". Although there were major differences between the regions, a large proportion of rural inhabitants only ate meat at Easter and to celebrate weddings. In 1888, about 50 % of the French population were farmers, whereas only 5 % of the population are farmers today.

The current boom in means of communication and the globalisation of exchanges have resulted in an abundance and diversity of foodstuffs, which have in turn led to an excess of food, a decrease in energy expenditure and an explosion in the frequency of obesity over the last two or three generations. How can we account for this abrupt change, when dietary habits have been changing for three or four generations in industrialised countries? A number of factors are probably involved, and these factors are likely to interact. However, several areas remain unclear: Whereas the amount of food eaten stopped increasing two or three decades ago, obesity is being detected increasingly early in children and affects an increasingly large proportion of the population, with a particularly marked increase in the number of severely obese individuals.

Genetics and obesity

The common forms involve several hundred genes that interact
with the environment

Classical Mendelian forms are rare: in very rare cases, obesity and diabetes can be considered to be monogenic hereditary diseases, in which only one gene is affected: LEPR, LEP, POMC, PCSK1, MC4R, SIMI1, UCP3, DRD4, GH and CART (obesity) INS, INRS, IRS1, NEUROD, PPARG, LMNA, HNF4A, GCK, HNF1A, IPF1 and HNF1B (diabetes).

However, the monogenic forms, which are often very severe, are very rare; in most cases, obesity and diabetes are multifactorial diseases (Fig. 2). Most cases

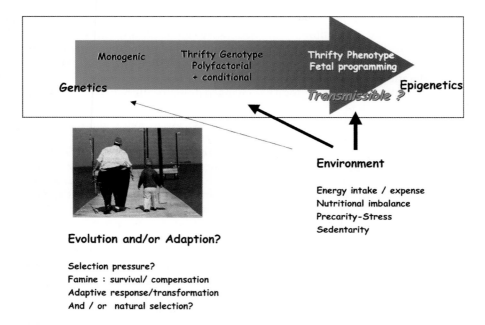

Fig. 2. The obesity epidemic: a blend of genetics, epigenetics and environment. The apparent obesity epidemic is not explained completely by increased food intake or decreased energy expenditure. Neither is it entirely explained by genetic background. In only a few cases of familial massive obesity, obesity can be considered a monogenic hereditary disease where one gene defect is sufficient. However, most cases are assumed to be multifactorial diseases: each individual has inherited a particular set of protective and deleterious alleles interacting with several environmental factors, including excess energy intake, lack of energy expenditure, and/or deleterious behaviors. According to the "thrifty genotype," first coined by JV Neel(1999), individuals living in an environment with unstable food supply could increase their probability of survival if they could maximize storage of surplus energy, for instance as abdominal fat. Repeated famines exert strong Darwinian selection pressure in favour of alleles of genes that can increase survival in cases of malnutrition. The repetition, intensity and duration of famines such as those that affected the Pima Indians (1870-1930), the Irish (1845-1849) or the Finnish (1866-1868) have led to the selection of more resistant individuals, those who were able to survive owing to thrifty genes. Conversely, during the nine months of siege at Amsterdam, Rotterdam and The Hague, although the rate of mortality did double, both adults and foetuses rapidly adapted in response to restrictions of calorie intake, without necessarily having to call upon thrifty genes. As an alternative to classical genetic mutations, epigenetic mechanisms resulting in changes in chromatin conformation, hence in alteration of the expression of genes, may be the cause of the "thrifty phenotype" observed in the Dutch subjected to the Dutch winter famine (Hales and Barker 1992).

correspond to multigene multifactorial forms, with each individual having inherited a particular set of susceptibility alleles and protective alleles for a number of genes, interacting with environmental and behavioural factors. The following susceptibility genes have been identified for diabetes: CETP, ABCC8 (SUR1), KCNJ11 (KIR6.2), PPARG, PGC1, HNF1A, PC-1, IRS1, CAPN10, VDR, LMNA, PON2, UCP1, UCP3; and the following susceptibility genes have been identified for obesity: MC4R, GNB3, CHE2, PPARG, ADRA2A, ADRB2, ADRB3, GR, FABP2, IGF1, UCP2-UCP3, BBS1, INS, LDLR, APOD, TNFA, LEPR, LEP, NMB, UCP1, SHP, etc. as well as several regions of the human or murine genome identified by whole genome analyses (Perusse et al. 2001). Twenty-four hereditary Mendelian disorders in which obesity is one of the main clinical manifestations have been identified, and in certain cases the genes involved have also been identified. The genes involved in the characteristic forms of these disorders may contribute to the common multigene forms via polymorphisms with less deleterious effects (Perusse et al. 2001).

The thrifty genotype

It is generally accepted that a particular molecular profile, "the thrifty genotype," which previously favoured a thrifty response to dietary restrictions, may account for the current explosion in obesity, in the context of dietary excess and a more sedentary way of life (Neel 1999).

This situation applies to the Pima Indians living in central Arizona and to the inhabitants of the Nauru Islands in the West Pacific. For other Indians from Canada, the Oji-Cree, the G319S mutation in the HNF-1a gene plays this role. In Caucasian populations, mutations in the melanocortin 4 receptor (MC4R) play this role (Cone 2000). Finally, in African and Asian populations, the GNB3-825T susceptibly allele is more frequent than in Caucasians (Gütersohn et al. l 2000). The term "thrifty genotype" has been used to describe many other genes (INS, APOE4, UCP1, PPARG, AGT, ADRB3, LPL, HSL, mtDNA, GYS, etc.).

However, this genetic model with strong selection pressure cannot account for the phenomenon of anticipation, i.e., the greater severity and earlier onset of obesity. Increasing numbers of transgenerational effects, not necessarily involving thrifty genotypes, have also been described.

Modifying genes, interaction of genes and environment

It is also clear that the phenotype of subjects carrying mutations responsible for monogenic diseases transmitted by classical Mendelian genetics may be variable. This variability is associated with allelic heterogeneity, environmental factors and/or modifying genes. These modifying genes may affect dominance, penetrance and pleiotropy.

Modifying genes, which may modulate response to a diet or a treatment, may also be subject to polymorphism. Polymorphism in these genes may result in considerable variation from one individual to the next. Although modifying genes are not directly responsible for the disease or the trait, they may trigger or interfere with the pathogenic process due to the existence of protective or deleterious alleles.

Unlike the alleles of predisposition or susceptibility genes, these protective or deleterious alleles are distributed similarly in affected subjects and controls. However, the frequency of the various alleles may differ between subjects with different subtypes of the disease. These alleles may affect the age at which the disease first appears, its severity or the organ affected (pleiotropy). The physiopathological consequences may become apparent only if the function of the modifier gene becomes critical, to compensate for the response to the endogenous substrate, a medicine or a food. Some subjects respond well, whereas others metabolise a substance much too rapidly (10 to 1000 times too rapidly), resulting in its inactivation; these subjects are not sensitive to this substance. Alternatively, the modifier gene may be subject to a conditional polymorphism, the effect of which is only detected in the presence of a specific environmental factor (G6PD and fava beans or primaquine).

A number of studies have addressed the role of gene-nutrient interactions in response to plasma lipid levels or nutrient variations in the dietary intake of fat or in response to calorie restriction. Polymorphisms have been identified in a large number of genes responsible for postprandial variability: APOA1, APOA2, APOA4, APOC3, APOE, APOB, HL, LPL, CETP, FABP2, FATP, PAI1, F7, MTHFR, ACE, PPPIR3; for variability in responses to a diet or a treatment: APOE, APOA1, APOA4, APOB, LPL, CETP, FABP2, MDR, FASN, PGC-1, PPARG, ADRB3, VDR, AT2R,1 HSD11B2, CYP11B2, ANP, ACE, AGT; and for variability in response to exercise: IGF1, LPL, GNB3, UCP1, UCP2-UCP3, LEP, ADRB2, ADRB1, ADRB3, ADRAB2, ANG, NOS3, CKMM, ATP1, APOE, TNFA, ACE, TGFB1, AGT, ACE, CYP11B2, etc. (Perusse et al. 2001).

Recently, much interest has been focused on the peroxisome proliferator-activated receptors (PPAR), which belong to the nuclear hormone receptor family of transcription factors. PPARG are involved in the differentiation of adipocytes. They also play a major role in type 2 diabetes and associated problems, such as insulin sensitivity, and the metabolism of lipids and energy. Numerous studies have been carried out to try to show that allele 12 Ala of PPARG has a protective effect against type 2 diabetes. Conflicting results have been obtained, depending on the populations studied. However, it is not impossible that the effect of this common variant is modified by diet. As the natural ligands of PPARG include fatty acids, the ratio of polyunsaturated to saturated fatty acids (P:S) may be involved. Recently, a study on a population of 592 non-diabetic subjects showed that, if P:S ratio was low, then BMI was higher in subjects carrying the Ala12 allele than in Pro/Pro homozygotes, but if P:S ratio was high, the inverse was true for subjects carrying the Ala12 allele. Similarly, allele Ala12 was not associated with high fasting insulinaemia if the P:S ratio was ≤ 0.39 quartile and the inverse was true if the P:S ratio was > 0.66 quartile. This gene/nutrient interaction is therefore limited to a single allele, the Ala12 allele of PPARG (Luan et al. 2001).

Epigenetics and obesity

The current situation may also result from modifications that appeared in our ancestors (grandparents) and were amplified before transmission to the current generation. Thus, could we be seeing not just a direct effect on individuals affected with obesity but also a progressive, transgenerational effect? The transmission of acquired traits to subsequent generations was long considered to be impossible, but it may in fact occur by epigenetic means. Epigenetic modifications that do not alter the DNA sequence, but are not erased during the passage through the germline, have been described in several species (Prak and Kazazian 2000). They may concern transposable elements and imprinted genes.

Epigenetic modifications of chromatin

Modifications of chromatin over time

Hereditary characteristics are transmitted by means of simple genetic information. However, diversification of the expression of the genetic material during development and in different tissues depends on epigenetic modifications, such as changes in DNA methylation and the structure of chromatin. Such changes alter the activity of the genome without changing the nucleotide sequence (Fig. 3). Although all the genes of an organism are transcribed during its life cycle, only a small proportion of these genes is required for differentiation into specialised cells. It is therefore essential for each cell type to select correctly the genes that should be switched on and those that should be switched off at a given moment. These mechanisms are disturbed in numerous disorders, including neurodegenerative diseases and tumours. The epigenetic mechanisms making it possible to establish tissue-specific expression during development require the resetting of the programme for the germline. These processes respond to dynamics controlled by parental, chromosomal and stage-specific factors. The process of methylation also has a fundamental role in embryo development as a whole (Fig. 3).

Functions of chromatin remodelling

Methylation is involved not only in the mechanisms governing the switching on and off of genes during cell differentiation but also in the fidelity of chromosomal segregation. Excluding the genes, 35 to 40 % of genomic DNA consists of repeated mobile elements present in multiple copies. These elements include a number of retroviral sequences that can move around autonomously. It is generally accepted that the methylation of these sequences comprises a host defence mechanism to limit the mobility of these sequences, which play an undeniable role in the process of evolution and in numerous physiopathological processes (e.g., cancer). In somatic cells, the hypomethylation of these sequences, frequently

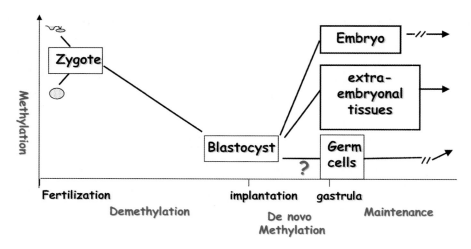

Fig. 3. Epigenetics : methylation, acetylation condensation, remodelling. As the first cell divisions occur, following the appearence of the first cell of the organism (the zygote), an intense wave of demethylation occurs, all «counters are set back to zero» except for imprinted genes which still carry the mark that will allow future cells to recognize their parental origin. After implantation and progressively through embryogenesis, a methylation program starts. This program will orient the expression or silencing of specific sets of genes to fulfill adequate differentiation processes for a given tissue or a given cell at the appropriate stage of development. Programming, deprogramming and reprogramming are therefore essential for proper development.

The methylation of a sequence triggers gene silencing, by recruiting a repressor complex, MBH/HDAC (methyl-binding domain/histone deacetylase), which alters the conformation of the chromatin and leads to the transient inactivation of gene expression. Stable repression is obtained by hypermethylation of the DNA, by a de novo-synthesised DNA methyl transferase, and supplementary remodelling of the DNA. This process may be carried out by the complexes involved in inactivation or by different complexes. To ensure that the inactivation is stable during cell division, the DNMT1 enzyme carries out maintenance methylation to ensure that the newly synthesised strand is identically methylated, and the MBD/HDAC complex remodels the chromatin. The inhibition of maintenance DNA methyl transferase activity, the action of a demethylase or inhibition of the deacetylase can lead to the demethylation, decondensation and derepression of inactive chromatin (Li 1999).

Methylation regulates the transcription of genes and therefore has a major effect on their expression. It acts as an epigenetic marker to enable regulation factors to distinguish between methylated sequences and identical non-methylated sequences. This process has a very important role in parental imprinting, the inactivation of the X chromosome in mammals and the repression of endogenous viruses

observed in tumour formation, favours mitotic recombination. Conversely, germline cells, which must undergo meiotic recombination, are hypomethylated.

Finally, methylation is involved in the differential marking of imprinted genes (IG). About 50 IG have already been identified in humans and mice. Our genome contains an estimated 100 to 200 IG (Morison and Reeve 1998). IG display monoallelic expression. Only the paternal or maternal allele is expressed, with the

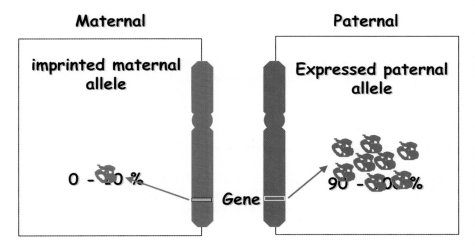

Maternal   **Paternal**

imprinted maternal allele

Expressed paternal allele

0 - 10 %

Gene

90 - 100 %

Fig. 4. Monoallelic expression of imprinted genes. About 50 imprinted genes have been identified in humans and mice. Our genome contains an estimated 100 to 200 imprinted genes (Morison and Reeve 1998). Imprinted genes, subject to parental or genomic imprinting, are characterised by monoallelic expression: according to the gene concerned, only the paternal allele or only the maternal allele is expressed (Robertson and Wolffe 2000).

other allele being affected by an epigenetic modification: chromatin condensation, deacetylation of histones and/or methylation (Robertson and Wolffe. 2000).

This is brought about by epigenetic instructions – imprints – that are laid down in the parental germ cells. It subsequently allows the transcriptional machinery to distinguish between the paternal and maternal chromosomes. However, it is clear that this imprint must be protected efficiently during the wave of demethylation that occurs in the zygote after fertilisation but before implantation (Fig. 4).

Thus, to explain the phenomenon of micro-evolution, it is possible that certain epigenetic "accidents" occur during the existence of an individual, for example, following exposure to stress. This does not explain how these DNA epimutations can be transmitted from an individual to his descendants, but this process probably involves an escape from the "reset function."

Epimutations and classical mutations

Epimutations present several advantages over classical mutations: they are more common, they can be targeted in a co-ordinated manner to several loci at once; their duration over time depends both on the genetic background and the epigenetic memory of the response, and they may be reversible. They have adjustable, quantitative effects and are probably less deleterious than classical mutations, which can alter the function of a gene. Furthermore, and in contrast with classical mutations, these epimutations can occur simultaneously in several individuals if these individuals are subjected to the same stimulus. A classical mutation or an epimutation can replicate in a clonal manner if it confers a selective advantage on the cell, possibly resulting in a tumour. A substance may be mutagenic for different sequences, by forming DNA adducts or by interfering with DNA repair or with the mechanisms responsible for epigenetic modifications.

Maternal effects

The "thrifty phenotype" hypothesis

Several maternal conditions are linked to obesity and affect the development of foetal neurones, both in humans and in rodents. Paradoxically, apparently contradictory situations, such as reduced calorie intake or maternal obesity, predispose the offspring to obesity. Similarly, mothers with type 1 or type 2 diabetes tend to have obese children. Finally, both excess food and the exposure of the newborns to exogenous insulin during the postnatal period lead to obesity. These apparently contradictory findings can be explained by the fact that these different types of perturbation affect the programming process at different times, inducing the so-called "thrifty phenotype" (Hales and Barker. 1992, 2001).

Several studies have shown that 1) type 2 diabetes is more often transmitted via the mother than via the father (Dorner and Mohnike 1976; Pettitt et al. 1987; Thomas et al. 1994), and 2) type 2 diabetes is more prevalent among children of mothers who were diabetic during their pregnancy than among children of non-diabetic or pre-diabetic mothers (Pettitt et al. 1987). Intra-uterine exposure to diabetes is also associated with a higher prevalence of glucose intolerance in adolescents (Silverman et al. 1995) and with a particularly striking excess obesity during the 20 first years of life (Pettitt et al. 1983). However, the effects of intra-uterine exposure to diabetes could be confounded by genetic factors. A recent study carried out on Pima Indians demonstrated that the risk of developing diabetes was higher in the children born after their mothers had developed diabetes (Dabelea et al. 2000; Fig. 5a). Intra-uterine growth retardation (IUGR) is also associated with the development of type 2 diabetes in adults rats (Simmons et al. 2000; Fig. 5b).

Neuronal "metabolic imprinting"

The epidemic of obesity in industrialised countries cannot be accounted for solely by the simultaneous increase in energy intake and decrease in energy expenditure. If genetically predisposed individuals become obese, their weight remains high even if they follow a strict, calorie-controlled diet. Genetically predisposed animals harbour numerous neuronal modifications that lead them to become obese when calorie intake increases. These abnormalities disappear when the individual becomes obese. This finding suggests that obesity is a "normal" state for these individuals. The formation of new neuronal circuits involved in the homeostasis of energy may account for the almost constant body weight. Such

a) Maternal diabetes

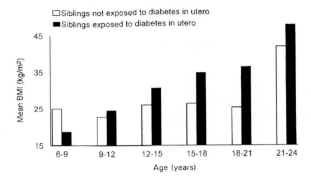

b) In utero denutrition

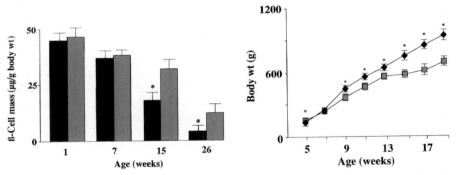

Fig. 5. Maternal effects. **a)** To discriminate between genetic factors and intrauterine exposure to diabetes, Dabelea et al. (2000) compared the prevalence of diabetes and BMI of Pima Indian children born before or after their mothers had developed diabetes. The risk of developing diabetes was higher in children born after their mothers had developed diabetes. And among nondiabetic children, the BMI was higher in those born to diabetic mothers. There were no differences in children born to diabetic fathers before or after the diagnosis of diabetes (Dabelea et al. 2000). **b)** Intrauterine growth retardation (IUGR) is linked to the development of type 2 diabetes in adults. Neonatal diabetes is also associated with IUGR (Marquis et al. 2000). Mechanisms involved are still unknown. Intrauterine growth retardation due to ligation of the uterine arteries in rats at the 19th day of gestation also leads to overt diabetes in adult rats. Diabetes is associated with a decline in beta cells of the pancreas (Simmons et al. 2001).

neuronal plasticity may exert its effects both during development and in adults (Levin 2000).

Maternal diabetes, obesity and undernutrition are associated with a risk of obesity in the children of these mothers and, particularly, in genetically predisposed individuals. A change in the neuronal circuits and their functioning frequently accompanies this type of obesity. This trend towards obesity can also be transmitted to subsequent generations by a process of forward leaking, an inevitable spiral in which weight increases from generation to generation. These data suggest a form of metabolic imprinting on the neuronal circuits involved in energy homeostasis in genetically predisposed individuals.

The drugs used to treat obesity, which act centrally, reduce the previously "protected" weight and modify the function of the neuronal pathways involved in energy homeostasis. However, they do not generally have a permanent effect on weight and neuronal function. Thus, the only means of preventing the formation of permanent neuronal connections capable of promoting and perpetuating obesity in genetically predisposed subjects may be to identify mothers, babies and adults predisposed to obesity as early as possible so that they can receive early treatment (Levin 2000).

Paternal effects

Disorders associated with altered expression of imprinted genes show a bias in parental transmission of the associated phenotype. Whereas maternal effects can be due either to alteration of imprinting or to maternal effects in utero, paternal effects can only be due to alteration of imprinted genes.

Children who inherit a paternal allele (INS VNTR Class I) associated with an increase in expression of the insulin gene in the foetal pancreas and of the IGF2 (insulin-like growth factor 2) gene in the placenta have a high risk of developing early obesity. The parental transmission of two alleles of a VNTR (variable number of tandem repeats) that regulates the expression of the insulin gene (INS) and of the insulin-like growth factor II (IGF2) gene results in skewed transmission. Indeed, children who inherit the class I allele from their father, but not from their mother, have an even greater risk (RR = 1.8) of developing early obesity than do those who inherit a class III allele.

The 11p15 region, which contains the INS and IGF2 genes, is imprinted. The imprinted gene IGF2 clearly shows monoallelic expression, limited to the paternal allele in virtually all tissues except the choroid plexus. Conversely, it is less clear in which tissues and at which stages of development the expression of the insulin gene is monoallelic and paternal. Only for the yolk sac is the situation clear: In this tissue, paternal, monoallelic expression has been clearly demonstrated in mice and humans (Moore et al. 2001). There is therefore still no explanation for this transmission bias. Given the frequency of this class I allele in the population, this risk affects 65–70 % of children. An increase in the expression of the paternal allele in utero due to the class I allele may predispose children to the accumulation of fat in the postnatal period (Le Stunff et al. 2001).

Transmission of acquired traits to subsequent generations

Transgenerational effects

Famines, foetal programming and transgenerational effects in humans

With 50 years of hindsight, we can now analyse the consequences on several generations of the drastic reduction in calorie intake in pregnant women during famines, such as those experienced during the Leningrad siege (1941-1944) or at the end of the Second World War at Rotterdam and The Hague in the Netherlands (October 1994 – May 1945; Grangé et al. 1999; Ravelli et al. 1998). The Dutch winter famine had a profound effect on the general health of what was otherwise a well-nourished population. In Amsterdam, the mortality rate in 1945 was more than double that of 1939, and it is likely that most of this increase in mortality was attributable to malnutrition and infections. However, women conceived and gave birth to babies, and it is in these babies (2414) that the effects of maternal malnutrition during different periods of gestation on health in adult life can be studied (Roseboom et al. 2001).

The effects of undernutrition depend upon its timing during gestation and the organs and systems developing during that critical time window (Fig. 6; Transgenerational inheritance: famine, undernutrition consequences). However, the relationship between fetal growth and obesity in later life is a complicated one. It is known that there is a very strong correlation between birth weight and the state of health in adults (type 2 diabetes, hypertension, obesity, hyperlipidaemia) and that this strong correlation can be accounted for by both genetic and non-genetic factors.

If foetal suffering, as reflected by a low birth weight, predisposes the infant to NIDDM, then there should be more cases of diabetes among Russians born during the Leningrad siege than in controls from the same region with the same genetic background who were not affected by the siege. This is not the case. One explanation could be that, contrary to the Dutch people, this Russian population was poorly nourished before and after the siege. This observation is consistent with the genetic hypothesis accounting for the link between birth weight and the risk of diabetes, hyperlipidaemia and hypertension, without any effect of dietary restrictions (Grangé et al. 1999). Conversely susceptibility to obesity seems to be linked to distress in utero. It seems that famine exposure in early gestation led to a disturbance of lipid metabolism, whereas in mid and late gestation it led to a disturbance of glucose insulin metabolism (Roseboom et al. 2001).

Effects on subsequent generations of disturbing neuroendocrine systems in young animals

How does this *adaptation* rather than *selection* pressure manifest itself? The possible role of epigenetic inheritance in transgenerational effects was suggested several years ago, but was not widely accepted as it was rapidly associated with a return to Lamarck's theories.

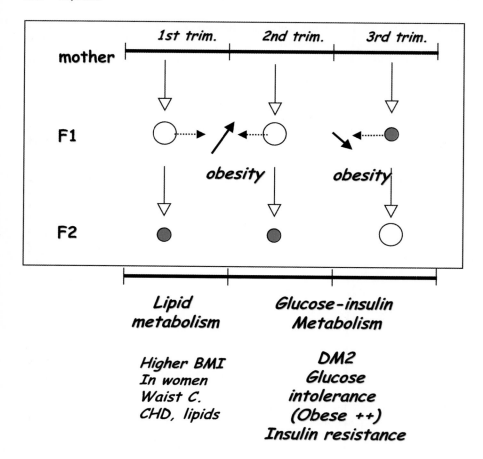

Transgenerational effects (TGE) have been observed in different species after exposure to various types of stimulus. Few transgenerational effects have been found in humans, but numerous experimental transgenerational effects related to treatments or deficiencies have been observed in animals. The observed effects occur after treatment with hormones (thyroid, parathyroid), the removal of the corresponding endocrine glands (pancreas, thyroid, parathyroid), the total or partial chemical destruction of the islets of Langerhans (insulin secretion), medical treatments (morphine), or dietary habits (betel nuts or dietary restrictions and glucose intolerance; Campbell and Perkins. 1988; Boucher et al. 1994; Jablonka et al. 1992).

Disturbances induced in the neuroendocrine systems of young treated animals may persist for long periods of time. The short-term effects are easier to examine but the changes that persist after discontinuation of the drug or changes in hormone levels are no less important. These effects extend beyond the strict limits of maternal effects on the foetus or of the tumorigenic effect of diethylstilboestrol on the daughters of treated mothers. The maternal effects are not hard to imag-

Fig. 6. Transgenerational inheritance: famine, undernutrition consequences. Children subjected to dietary restrictions in utero during the third trimester of pregnancy had lower birth weights (6 to 10 % lower than the birth weights recorded before the famine), due to a direct effect of the mothers' dietary restrictions on the foetus. Foetuses exposed to dietary restrictions have an increased risk of glucose intolerance, insulin resistance, obesity and type 2 diabetes. This is probably due to disruption of the programming of endocrine systems (Hales and Barker 1992) and of key centres of the central nervous system (Levin 2000). A study of 702 subjects born between 1/11/43 and 28/2/47 showed an increase in fasting insulin concentration and insulin concentration two hours after glucose ingestion for those exposed during the last semester (Ravelli et al. 1998). Glucose tolerance was decreased most among participants who were exposed during mid or late gestation. The effect on glucose tolerance is especially important in people who became obese. Maternal malnutrition during early gestation was associated with higher BMI and waist circumference in 50-year-old women but not in men (Ravelli et al. 1999). Thus maternal malnutrition during gestation may permanently affect adult health without affecting the size of the baby. Children who were subject to dietary restrictions in utero during the first semester of pregnancy had similar birth weights to other newborns. However, in spite of these normal birth weights, a higher incidence of obesity was observed in adult subjects (50-year-old women) of the first generation exposed to dietary restriction during the first semester of pregnancy. Surprisingly, the second generation, i.e., the children born to these subjects between 1960 and 1987, had lower birth weights (50-100 g below average). The reduced birth weight of these babies whose grandmothers suffered acute starvation in mid-pregnancy supports the action of transgenerational adaption to nutrition (Lumey 1992; Martin et al. 2000; Ravelli et al. 1998).

---

ine. However, the effects that persist in grandchildren or in great-grandchildren are considerably more surprising. In particular, these effects occur in the absence of a stimulus, not only through the maternal line but also, unexpectedly, through the paternal line, and affect several generations (Belyaev et al. 1981; Boucher et al. 1994; Jablonka et al. 1992; Martin et al. 2000).

In animals, transgenerational effects have been observed in a large number of studies (Belyaev et al.,1981; Boucher et al. 1994; Campbell and Perkins 1988; Jablonka et al. 1992). Eight of the nine groups who treated animals (rats, guinea pigs and rabbits) with diabetes-inducing drugs, such as alloxan, observed this type of effect. The F1 animals had fewer beta cells and the pituitary and adrenal glands were also affected. If the F1 animals were in turn treated with alloxan, the number of beta cells decreased further. Diabetes occurred in the F5 generation if the mothers and fathers were treated in each generation, and in the F7 generation if only the fathers were treated. Pancreatectomy in six generations of female rats led to glucose intolerance in the F7 generation. In another study, subdiabetogenic amounts of alloxan were injected into one generation of rats before weaning and these animals were crossed with each other and with control subjects. The offspring resulting from crossing the treated males with normal females showed significantly lower levels of glucose tolerance than did the offspring of other crosses. The F1 generation was pooled and the animals were crossed with each other for six generations without further treatment. The level of glucose tolerance progressively decreased. Some rats from the fifth generation were diabetic and others were unusually sensitive to alloxan. Thus consequences of the treatment of males crossed with normal females can be observed in the descendants several generations after the treatment (Campbell and Perkins. 1988).

Some of the consequences of the famines observed in humans at the end of the last world war have been confirmed by experimental data in rats (Martin et al. 2000; Ravelli et al. 1998). Studies reproducing these situations have been carried out in a number of animals (Belyaev et al. 1981; Boucher et al. 1994; Jablonka *et al.* 1992; Martin et al. 2000). Recently, pregnant female rats were fed with a low-protein diet. The F1 generation was fed normally, but nonetheless 30 % less insulin was secreted in response to glucose ingestion. Although the animals of the F1 generation were fed normally, the amount of insulin secreted increased by 80 % in the F2 generation. This increase was even greater (130 %) if the F1 generation was fed a fat-rich diet. Thus, in the second generation, a transgenerational effect of the low-protein diet was observed and hyperinsulinaemia was accentuated if fat intake was high (Martin et al. 2000). This animal model seems to reproduce the characteristics of the current obesity epidemic.

A known transmission medium: mobile elements/transposons

The total rejection of Lamarck's theories probably led us to neglect such observations, for which were therefore formulated explanations often described as heretical.

Transposable elements become methylated

Transposable elements (mobile sequences or transposons), which are DNA sequences that are able to move from one chromosomal site to another, account for 35–40 % of the human genome. The movement of transposable elements may cause structural or functional changes in the genome and may favour the installation of certain epigenetic regulatory mechanisms. About 10 % of mouse mutants involve the insertion of a transposon into a gene. The degree to which a transposon is methylated may alter the expression of the gene into which it is inserted (Robertson 1996).

Maternal transmission of epigenetic alterations

A mechanism for this type of epigenetic transmission was recently described for the *agouti* locus (A) in mice (Morgan et al. 1999 ; Fig. 7). Changes in the fur colour and other phenotypic aspects depend on the methylation of a transposable IAP sequence inserted close to gene A. The variable phenotypes observed in the offspring are due to the incomplete erasure of the epigenetic modification when allele A is transmitted via the maternal germ line (Whitelaw and Martin. 2001).

Although it is tempting to accept this model, the random movements of transposons cannot account for the rapid effects, almost identical in different subjects, of recent mutations, which appeared rapidly due to the amount and nature of food available and the degree of activity of the individuals (Whitelaw and Martin. 2001). Morever, random transposon movements cannot account for the increas-

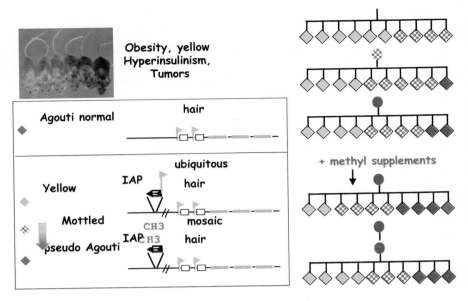

Fig. 7. Agouti locus: methylation and transposon. Epigenetic alterations that may not be completely erased through germline are now described in several species. They affect transposable elements and imprinted genes. Insertion of a transposon within a gene is responsible for about 10 % of mouse mutants. Epigenetic inheritance through the germline has recently been demonstrated in viable, Avy yellow mice in which insertion of a retrotransposon upstream of the Agouti gene (A) results in ectopic expression of agouti protein with a characteristic phenotype of yellow fur, obesity, diabetes and an increased incidence of tumors. However, there is a great variability in the phenotype of the offspring due to silencing of the transposon by methylation. The phenotype shows extremely variable expressivity in isogenic mice and is linked to activity of the inserted retrotransposon. Silencing in the offspring depends on the level of silencing of the IAP sequence in the mother and can be modified by feeding the mother with adequate levels of methyl **donnors**. The maternal phenotype is partially heritable, ranging from activity in nearly all cells to activity in only scattered cells (Whitelaw and Martin 2001).

ing number of transgenerational effects, which are often associated with skewed parental transmission.

An ideal candidate: parental or genomic imprinting

Conversely, thanks to the flexibility of rapid and reversible epigenetic modifications, genomic or parental imprinting may provide the logistic means required for a species to adapt to its environment in response to a given stimulus (Junien 2000; Pembrey 1996).

Imprinting and fluctuations in monoallelic expression

According to M. Pembrey, "the nature of imprinted genes poised, as it were, between a transcriptionally active and silent state makes them good candidates for incorporation into the evolution of transgenerational adaption systems where coordinated changes in gene expression are a selective advantage. Genomic imprinting as we observe it now could in fact just be a phase in a slow drift into transcriptional silence." It remains theoretically possible that changes in the level of transcriptional regulators in the germline, gamete or zygote could modify the setting of the imprint. In somatic cells transcriptional regulators can induce sequence specific demethylation or modify chromatin structure. There are several examples of functional polymorphisms: while monoallelic expression of IGF2R is found in only 10 % of individuals, all mouse strains examined showed monoallelic expression of this maternally expressed gene. In addition, the active allele might become silent or its transcription might stop earlier in one species or be limited to some tissues. This is what is observed for IGF2. It is possible that changing circumstances over several generations might recruit them back into the active genome and account for the reversibility of these adaptive changes (Pembrey 1996; Junien 2000; Fig. 8).

Diabetes and obesity and imprinted genes

In humans, as well as in mice, defects in the mechanisms of parental imprinting, in their erasure and in switching (changes as a function of sex) are associated with various syndromes [e.g., Prader Willi syndrome (PWS), Beckwith-Wiedemann syndrome (BWS), Albright Hereditary Osteodystrophy (AHO), Silver-Russel (SR), neonatal diabetes (DNN)], the symptoms of which may include intrauterine growth retardation, hypothyroidism, obesity or being underweight. Diabetes and obesity often accompany the syndromes associated with altered imprinting (Tilghman 1999).

Of the six loci encoding quantitative traits (QTL) affecting the body composition of the pig, five, including the IGF2 gene, are imprinted. These QTL affect the skeletal and cardiac muscular masses, the thickness of fat on the back, the depth of muscles and the fat content of muscles (Rattink et al. 2000).

Brain development and imprinted genes

Imprinted genes also play an important role in the development of the brain (Junien 2000; Keverne 2001). The analysis of chimeric mice, containing a certain amount of parthenogenetic and androgenetic cells, made it possible to follow the effects of IG on the development of the brain. At birth, the cells disomic for the paternal genome (androgenetic) contribute considerably to the development of the hypothalamus, septum, pre-optic area and basal nucleus of the stria terminalis, but these cells cannot survive in the developing neocortex or in the striatum. Conversely, the cells disomic for the maternal genome (gynogenetic) multi-

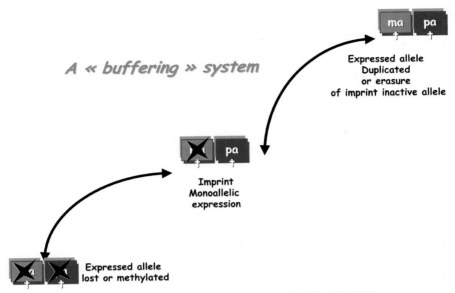

A « buffering » system

Expressed allele
Duplicated
or erasure
of imprint inactive allele

Imprint
Monoallelic
expression

Expressed allele
lost or methylated

Pembrey M. Acta Genet Med Gemellol 1996

Fig. 8. Genomic imprinting: variations, polymorphisms, plasticity. Monoallelic expression of imprinted gene may differ (becoming biallelic, for example) between species, between individuals and between tissues (Sakatani et al. 2001). IG may play a role in transgenerational adaptation processes in response to the environment. The flexibility of rapid and reversible epigenetic modifications may also make parental imprinting the ideal logistical means for the adaptation of a species to its environment. According to this hypothesis, parental imprinting, an epigenetic support for TGE, may facilitate rapid but also reversible adaptation to the environment (Pembrey 1996; Whitelaw and Martin 2001). ma, maternal ; pat, paternal.

ply in the cortex and in the striatum but are excluded from diencephalic structures. Two paternally expressed IG, *Mest* and *Peg3*, are strongly expressed in the regions in which androgenetic cells accumulate: the hypothalamus, pre-optic area and septum. Given the key role of the neurones of the hypothalamus in the regulation of energy homeostasis (hunger/satiety, intake of food or stopping eating), these genes may play a role in the neuronal programming mechanisms proposed by B.E. Levin (2000). The disruption of their monoallelic expression may be responsible for abnormal growth of these structures.

Interaction of environmental and epigenetic factors: folate intake during pregnancy

In the mouse, diet, especially folate intake, during the gestation period affects methylation. If the mother's diet is rich in methyl donors, the proportion of variable phenotypes of the viable yellow mutant at the *agouti* A^{vy} locus is altered. As already mentionned data have shown that variability in phenotypic expression is linked to the repression by methylation of a transposon-like sequence inserted upstream from the *agouti* gene (Whitelaw and Martin .2001). However, we still do not know whether epigenetic modifications linked to environmental factors can be transmitted to subsequent generations (Wolff et al. 1998).

A maternal diet low in protein during the gestation period is associated with changes in glucose tolerance and hypertension in the offspring. Threonine supplements (the only essential amino acid for which concentration decreases dramatically) lead to an increase in serum homocysteine concentration, accompanied by changes in the methylation status of hepatic DNA. An increase in maternal homocysteine levels may compromise foetal development, leading to glucose intolerance and hypertension (Rees et al. 2000).

Reconciling Lamarck and Darwin?

The transmission of transgenerational effects over several generations would also reopen the debate about the inheritance of acquired characteristics, a sort of "pseudo-Lamarckism." This may stimulate the long debate on the inheritance of acquired characteristics proposed almost two centuries ago by J.B Lamarck but strongly criticised later by A. Weismann (1834–1914). Whatever the nature of the epigenetic medium responsible for transgenerational effects, it may provide a means of rapidly adapting to changes in resources (obesity, diabetes), various types of aggression (immune response, allergies) or climatic changes so as to increase the survival capacities of both the individual and the whole species. These epimutations enable the species to adapt rapidly to its environment, without having to wait for Darwinian mutation. This is particularly true as methylation can be reversible, meaning that after a couple of generations the species may revert to its previous state. Interestingly, the methylation involved in the epimutation may also favour the appearance of real mutation by deamination of a methylcytosine leading to thymine (C'T). A gene methylated in this way would have a greater probability of permanent alteration if environmental pressure maintained the epimutation in a large number of generations.

Acquired traits would thus have an evolutionary value. These environmental changes could result from climatic changes, changes in hygiene conditions and in stress or qualitative and quantitative changes in diet. Although the available data are incomplete, the relevance of the questions addressed increases the value of studying transgenerational effects (Campbell and Perkins. 1988; Jablonka et al. 1992).

The *explosion* in obesity may also be slowed down by epigenetic resistance. There is nothing to stop us thinking that the current environment (leading to the prompt development of excess weight) can provoke insensitive traumatisms causing specific epimutations and changes in chromatin structure in many individuals. These changes may then be transmitted to future generations, thanks to parental imprinting in the gametes, and may indicate to the developing organism (the future child) that the environment has changed to such an extent that weight maintenance mechanisms should be modified.

This process is essentially the inverse process to that affecting the grandchildren of women who were severely deprived of food during the Stalingrad siege or at the end of the Second World War in Europe. Instead of "making more fat" than normal, due to the epigenetic "memory" of the famines experienced by their grandparents, the children and grandchildren of obese families may occasionally be of normal weight despite having an unfavourable genetic background (by definition) and an equally hostile mode of life (similar to that of their forefathers) due to modifications of the organism better able to "juggle" with excess calories and a lack of energy expenditure.

Abbreviations

ABCC8 ATP-BINDING CASSETTE, SUBFAMILY C, MEMBER 8,
ACE ANGIOTENSIN CONVERTING ENZYME,
ADM ADRENOMEDULLIN,
ADRA2A ALPHA-2A-ADRENERGIC RECEPTOR,
ADRA2B ALPHA-2B-ADRENERGIC RECEPTOR,
ADRB1 BETA-1-ADRENERGIC RECEPTOR,
ADRB2 BETA-2-ADRENERGIC RECEPTOR,
ADRB3 BETA-3-ADRENERGIC RECEPTOR,
AGT ANGIOTENSIN I,
AGTR1 ANGIOTENSIN RECEPTOR 1,
AHO Albright hereditary osteodystrophy,
ANG ANGIOGENIN,
ANP ATRIAL NATRIURIC PEPTIDE PRECURSOR,
APOA1 APOLIPOPROTEIN A-I,
APOA2 APOLIPOPROTEIN A-II,
APOA4 APOLIPOPROTEIN A-IV,
APOB APOLIPOPROTEIN B,
APOC3 APOLIPOPROTEIN C-III,
APOD APOLIPOPROTEIN D,
APOE APOLIPOPROTEIN E,
APOE4 APOLIPOPROTEIN E-IV,
AT2R1 ANGIOTENSIN II RECEPTOR, VASCULAR TYPE 1,
ATP1, SODIUM POTASSIUM ATPase,
BBS1 BARDET-BIEDL SYNDROME 1,
BWS Beckwith-Wiedemann syndrome,
CAPN10 CALPAIN 10,
CART COCAINE- AND AMPHETAMINE-REGULATED TRANSCRIPT,
CETP CHOLESTEROL ESTER TRANSFER PROTEIN,
CHE2 CHOLINESTERASE, SERUM, 2,
CKMM CREATINE KINASE M,
CYP11B2 CYTOCHROME P450, SUBFAMILY XIB, POLYPEPTIDE 2,
DNMT1 DNA METHYLTRANSFERASE 1,
DNN Neonatal diabetes,
DRD4 DOPAMINE RECEPTOR D4,

EDN1 ENDOTHELIN 1,
F7 COAGULATION FACTOR VII,
FABP2 FATTY ACID BINDING PROTEIN-2,
FASN FATTY ACID SYNTHASE,
FGFR3 FIBROBLAST GROWTH FACTOR RECEPTOR 3,
G6PD GLUCOSE-6-PHOSPHATE DEHYDROGENASE,
GCK GLUCOKINASE,
GH, Ghrelin
GNB3 GUANINE NUCLEOTIDE-BINDING PROTEIN, BETA-3,
GYS1 GLYCOGEN SYNTHASE 1,
HL or HTGL HEPATIC TRIGLYCERIDE LIPASE,
HNF1A or HNF-1-ALPHA HEPATIC NUCLEAR FACTOR-1-ALPHA,
HNF1B or HNF-1-BETA HEPATIC NUCLEAR FACTOR-1-BETA,
HNF4A HEPATOCYTE NUCLEAR FACTOR 4-ALPHA,
HSD11B2 CORTISOL 11-BETA-KETOREDUCTASE,
HSL or LIPE LIPASE HORMONE-SENSITIVE,
IG Imprinted gene,
IGF1 INSULIN LIKE GROWTH FACTOR 1,
IGF2 INSULIN LIKE GROWTH FACTOR 2,
IGF2R INSULIN-LIKE GROWTH FACTOR 2 RECEPTOR,
INS INSULIN,
INSR INSULIN RECEPTOR,
IPF1 INSULIN PROMOTER FACTOR 1,
IRS1 INSULIN RECEPTOR SUBSTRATE 1,
IUGR Intra-uterine growth retardation
KCNJ11 POTASSIUM CHANNEL, INWARDLY RECTIFYING, SUBFAMILY J,
    MEMBER 11,
LDLR LOW DENSITY LIPOPROTEIN RECEPTOR,
LEP LEPTIN,
LEPR LEPTIN RECEPTOR,
LMNA LAMIN A/C,
LPL LIPOPROTEIN LIPASE,
MC4R MELANOCORTIN 4 RECEPTOR,
MDR MULTI DRUG RESISTANCE,
MEST MESODERM-SPECIFIC TRANSCRIPT, MOUSE, HOMOLOG OF,
MTHFR METHYLENE TETRAHYDROFOLATE REDUCTASE I,
MYO9A MYOSIN IXA
NDN NECDIN,
NEUROD NEUROGENIC DIFFERENTIATION,
NIDDM DIABETES MELLITUS, NONINSULIN-DEPENDENT,
NMB NEUROMEDIN B,
NOS3 NITRIC OXIDE SYNTHASE 3,
PC1 PROPROTEIN CONVERTASE 1,
PCSK1 PROPROTEIN CONVERTASE, SUBTILISIN/KEXIN-TYPE, 1,
PEG3 PATERNALLY EXPRESSED GENE 3,
PGC-1 PEROXISOME PROLIFERATOR ACTIVATED-RECEPTOR-GAMMA
    COACTIVATOR,

PIA1 PLASMINOGEN ACTIVATOR INHIBITOR, TYPE 1,FATP FATTY ACID
   TRANSPORT PROTEINS,
POMC PROOPIOMELANOCORTIN,
PON2 PARAOXONASE 2,
PPARG PEROXISOME PROLIFERATOR-ACTIVATED RECEPTOR-GAMMA,
PPPIR3 PROTEIN PHOSPHATASE 1,
PWS Prader-Willi syndrome,
QTL Quantitative traits loci
SCNN1G (SCNEG) SODIUM CHANNEL, NONVOLTAGE-GATED 1, GAMMA
   SUBUNIT (SODIUM CHANNEL, EPITHELIAL, GAMMA SUBUNIT),
SHP SMALL HETERODIMER PARTNER
SIMI1 SINGLE MINDED (DROSOPHILA) HOMOLOG 1,
SNRPN SMALL NUCLEAR RIBONUCLEOPROTEIN POLYPEPTIDE N,
SR Silver-Russel,
TBX3 T-BOX 3,
TGE Transgenerational effects
TGFB1 TRANSFORMING GROWTH FACTOR 1,
THRB THYROID HORMONE RECEPTOR, BETA,
TNFA TUMOR NECROSIS FACTOR ALPHA,
UCP1 UNCOUPLING PROTEIN 1,
UCP2 UNCOUPLING PROTEIN 2,
UCP3 UNCOUPLING PROTEIN 3,
VDR VITAMIN D RECEPTOR,
VNTR Variable number of tandem repeat,

EDNRA ENDOTHELIN RECEPTOR, TYPE A
Alternative titles; symbols
ETRA (ETA) ENDOTHELIN RECEPTOR, ET1-SPECIFIC TYPE,

References

Belyaev DK, Ruvinsky AO, Borodin PM (1981) Inheritance of alternative states of the fused gene
   in mice. J Hered 72: 107-112.
Boucher BJ, Ewen SW, Stowers JM (1994) Betel nut (Areca catechu) consumption and the induc-
   tion of glucose intolerance in adult CD1 mice and in their F1 and F2 offspring [see com-
   ments]. Diabetologia 37: 49-55.
Campbell JH, Perkins P (1988) Transgenerational effects of drug and hormonal treatments in
   mammals: a review of observations and ideas. Prog Brain Res 73: 535-553.
Cone RD (2000) Haploinsufficiency of the melanocortin-4 receptor: part of a thrifty genotype?
   J Clin Invest 106: 185-187.
Dabelea D, Hanson RL, Lindsay RS, Pettitt DJ, Imperatore G, Gabir MM, Roumain J, Bennett PH,
   Knowler WC (2000) Intrauterine exposure to diabetes conveys risks for type 2 diabetes and
   obesity: a study of discordant sibships. Diabetes 49: 2208-2211.
Dorner G, Mohnike A (1976) Further evidence for a predominantly maternal transmission of
   maturity-onset type diabetes. Endokrinologie 68: 121-124.
Grangé G, Dupont J-M, Jeanpierre M (1999) Gènes et retards de croissance intra-utérins. Méd
   Sci 15: 82-85.

Gütersohn A, Mueller R, Siffert W (2000). The GNB3 825T-allele is associated with obesity. Support for the thrifty genotype hypothesis.Circulation 102: II-849.

Hales CN, Barker DJ (1992) Type 2 (non-insulin-dependent) diabetes mellitus: the thrifty phenotype hypothesis. Diabetologia 35: 595-601.

Hales CN, Barker DJ (2001) The thrifty phenotype hypothesis. Brit Med Bull 60: 5-20.

Jablonka E, Lachmann M, Lamb MJ (1992) Evidence, mechanisms and models for the inheritance of acquired charaters. J Theoret Biol 158: 245-268.

Junien C (2000) L'empreinte parentale: de la guerre des sexes à la solidarité entre générations. Méd Sci 3: 336-344.

Keverne E (2001) Genomic imprinting and the maternal brain. Prog Brain Res 133: 279-285.

Le Stunff C, Fallin D, Bougneres P (2001) Paternal transmission of the very common class I INS VNTR alleles predisposes to childhood obesity. Nat Genet 29: 96-99.

Levin BE (2000) The obesity epidemic: metabolic imprinting on genetically susceptible neural circuits. Obes Res 8: 342-347.

Li E (1999) The mojo of methylation. Nature Genet 23: 5-6.

Luan J, Browne PO, Harding AH, Halsall DJ, O'Rahilly S, Chatterjee VK, Wareham NJ (2001) Evidence for gene-nutrient interaction at the PPARgamma locus. Diabetes 50: 686-689.

Lumey LH (1992) Decreased birthweights in infants after maternal in utero exposure to the Dutch famine of 1944-1945. Paediatr Perinat Epidemiol 6: 240-253.

Marquis E, Robert JJ, Benezech C, Junien C, Diatloff-Zito C (2000) Variable features of transient neonatal diabetes mellitus with paternal isodisomy of chromosome 6. Eur J Human Genet 8: 137-140.

Martin JF, Johnston CS, Han CT, Benyshek DC (2000) Nutritional origins of insulin resistance: a rat model for diabetes- prone human populations. J Nutr 130: 741-744.

Moore GE, Abu-Amero SN, Bell G, Wakeling EL, Kingsnorth A, Stanier P, Jauniaux E, Bennett ST (2001) Evidence that insulin is imprinted in the human yolk sac. Diabetes 50: 199-203.

Morgan HD, Sutherland HG, Martin DI, Whitelaw E (1999) Epigenetic inheritance at the agouti locus in the mouse. Nature Genet 23: 314-318.

Morison IM, Reeve AE (1998) A catalogue of imprinted genes and parent-of-origin effects in humans and animals. Human Mol Genet 7: 1599-1609.

Neel JV (1999) Diabetes mellitus: a "thrifty" genotype rendered detrimental by "progress"? 1962. Bull World Health Org 77: 694-703.

Pembrey M (1996) Imprinting and transgenerational modulation of gene expression; human growth as a model. Acta Genet Med Gemellol 45: 111-125.

Perusse L, Chagnon YC, Weisnagel SJ, Rankinen T, Snyder E, Sands J, Bouchard C (2001) The human obesity gene map: the 2000 update. Obes Res 9: 135-169.

Pettitt DJ, Baird HR, Aleck KA, Bennett PH, Knowler WC (1983) Excessive obesity in offspring of Pima Indian women with diabetes during pregnancy. New Engl J Med 308: 242-245.

Pettitt DJ, Knowler WC, Bennett PH, Aleck KA, Baird HR (1987) Obesity in offspring of diabetic Pima Indian women despite normal birth weight. Diabetes Care 10: 76-80.

Prak ET, Kazazian HH, Jr. (2000) Mobile elements and the human genome. Nat Rev Genet 1: 134-144.

Rattink AP, De Koning DJ, Faivre M, Harlizius B, van Arendonk JA, Groenen MA (2000) Fine mapping and imprinting analysis for fatness trait QTLs in pigs. Mamm Genome 11: 656-661.

Ravelli AC, van der Meulen JH, Michels RP, Osmond C, Barker DJ, Hales CN, Bleker OP (1998) Glucose tolerance in adults after prenatal exposure to famine. Lancet 351: 173-177.

Ravelli AC, van Der Meulen JH, Osmond C, Barker DJ, Bleker OP (1999) Obesity at the age of 50 y in men and women exposed to famine prenatally. Am J Clin Nutr 70: 811-816.

Rees WD, Hay SM, Brown DS, Antipatis C, Palmer RM (2000) Maternal protein deficiency causes hypermethylation of DNA in the livers of rat fetuses. J Nutr 130: 1821-1826.

Robertson HM (1996) Members of the pogo superfamily of DNA-mediated transposons in the human genome. Mol Gen Genet 252: 761-766.

Robertson KD, Wolffe AP (2000) DNA methylation in health and disease. Nature Rev Genet 1: 11-19.

Roseboom TJ, van der Meulen JH, van Montfrans GA, Ravelli AC, Osmond C, Barker DJ, Bleker OP (2001) Maternal nutrition during gestation and blood pressure in later life. J Hypertens 19: 29-34.

Sakatani T, Wei M, Katoh M, Okita C, Wada D, Mitsuya K, Meguro M, Ikeguchi M, Ito H, Tycko B, Oshimura M (2001) Epigenetic heterogeneity at imprinted loci in normal populations. Biochem Biophys Res Commun 283: 1124-1130.

Silverman BL, Metzger BE, Cho NH, Loeb CA (1995) Impaired glucose tolerance in adolescent offspring of diabetic mothers. Relationship to fetal hyperinsulinism. Diabetes Care 18: 611-617.

Simmons RA, Templeton LJ, Gertz SJ (2001) Intrauterine growth retardation leads to the development of type 2 diabetes in the rat. Diabetes 50: 2279-2286.

Thomas F, Balkau B, Vauzelle-Kervroedan F, Papoz L (1994) Maternal effect and familial aggregation in NIDDM. The CODIAB Study. CODIAB-INSERM-ZENECA Study Group. Diabetes 43: 63-67.

Tilghman SM (1999) The sins of the fathers and mothers: genomic imprinting in mammalian development. Cell 96: 185-193.

Whitelaw E, Martin DI (2001) Retrotransposons as epigenetic mediators of phenotypic variation in mammals. Nature Genet 27: 361-365.

Wolff GL, Kodell RL, Moore SR, Cooney CA (1998) Maternal epigenetics and methyl supplements affect agouti gene expression in Avy/a mice. Faseb J 12: 949-957.

Subject Index

Printing: Mercedes-Druck, Berlin
Binding: Stein+Lehmann, Berlin